THE LEGEND OF THE
DEATH RACE

Conquering Life with

Courage, Power, & Wisdom

Foreword By Joe De Sena

As Told By
Tony Matesi

UP, BEYOND PUBLISHING

This book is a memoir. It reflects the author's recollections of these experiences over time. Some names and characteristics have been changed, some events have been compressed, and some dialogue has been recreated. The author consulted with other Death Racers to keep the story as true to how it happened as they collectively remember it.

The Legend of the Death Race
Copyright © 2020 by Legend of the Death Race, LLC

Trademarks belong to their respective owners.

Spartan Race, and Death Race, and their respective logos, are trademarks of Spartan Race, Inc.

Published in Seattle, WA in the United States by Up, Beyond Publishing, a division of Up Beyond Media, LLC.
www.upbeyondmedia.com.

Cover Illustration by Ella Anne Kociuba

All rights reserved. No part of this book may be reproduced or used in any manner without the written permission of the copyright owner except for the use of quotations in a book review. For more information, address: www.legendofthedeathrace.com

FIRST EDITION
www.legendofthedeathrace.com

Library of Congress Cataloging in Publication Data
Names: Matesi, Tony, Author. De Sena, Joe, Foreword. Title: The Legend of the Death Race: Conquering Life with Courage, Power, & Wisdom / by Tony Matesi
Other Titles: The Legend of the Death Race
Description: First Edition. | Seattle, WA : Up, Beyond Publishing, 2020.

Identifiers: LCCN 2020902597 | ISBN: 978-1-7345417-1-7 (hardcover) | ISBN: 978-1-7345417-2-4 (audio) | ISBN: 978-1-7345417-0-0 (paperback) | ISBN: 978-1-7345417-3-1 (ebook)

For my parents, Rich and Darnell, who taught me to always seek the best for myself, to forever be courageous, and to never settle for mediocrity.

In Loving Memory of Todd Schwartz, your encouragement and ability to see what I sometimes could not see in myself is what fueled me to complete this memoir.

Thank you for always believing in me.

You were the mentor I needed.

CONTENTS

Foreword By: Joe De Sena - Founder Of The Death Race 1

Prologue - Before Death..5

YEAR 1 - COURAGE

Chapter 1 - Destination: Death Race, Vermont............................ 10

Chapter 2 - The Beginning 14

Chapter 3 - Crawling Under Highways, Pink Swim Caps And Slosh Pipes...20

Chapter 4 - Bloodroot 27

Chapter 5 - The Tribulations Of Team Tire 35

Chapter 6 - Human Error Or Betrayal 42

Chapter 7 - Make It Hurt So Good 51

Chapter 8 - The Comeback Kids...59

Chapter 9 - And We'll Keep Fighting Til The End 66

Chapter 10 - Sleepyhead 75

Chapter 11 - Never Quit, Never Surrender..................................81

Chapter 12 - The Months After Death 92

YEAR 2 - POWER

Chapter 13 - Jet-Setter..100

Chapter 14 - Stairway To Heaven 107

Chapter 15 - Mile High Staircase..112

Chapter 16 - Ready, Set... 119

Chapter 17 - A Dance With Barbed Wire 129

Chapter 18 - The Unexpected 136

Chapter 19 - Between A Rock And A Hard Place: Bloodroot ..144

Chapter 20 - Surviving The Delusions 151

Chapter 21 - Down With The Sickness... 157

Chapter 22 - Swim To Death... 163

Chapter 23 - The Spartan Life..171

YEAR 3 - WISDOM

Chapter 24 - Here We Go Again...178

Chapter 25 - Another Beginning... 186

Chapter 26 - Return Of The Stone Stairs.................................195

Chapter 27 - Bloodroot Water Giver.. 201

Chapter 28 - Pocahontas And Porcupine Quills....................... 208

Chapter 29 - Charred Axes And A Bucket Full Of Lies..............215

Chapter 30 - A Ravine And A Cemetery 222

Chapter 31 - Endless Yoga 227

Chapter 32 - Comin' In Hot..236

Chapter 33 - A Tale Of Two Buses 244

Chapter 34 - The Final Hours 252

Chapter 35 - Skulls 259

Epilogue 271

Acknowledgments 274

Glossary 278

About The Author 283

FOREWORD

BY JOE DE SENA
FOUNDER OF THE DEATH RACE & SPARTAN RACE

Suffering is an authentic part of the human experience. But a form of sport?

The first time I saw it that way, I was a teenager living in Queens, NY, in the 1980s. My mother Jean and I went to watch what is now known as the Self-Transcendence 3,100 Mile Race that was happening in the borough. It's an insane race: People run around a 1-mile loop from 6 AM to midnight for 52 straight days, totaling 3,100 miles. It's the world's longest certified road race, now in its 23rd year.

I remember watching those runners and wondering, "Wow, what is a human being capable of? And what motivates someone to test himself like this?"

It was a watershed moment for me, even though I wasn't a runner. At that young age, business was my sport. I just wanted to make money. But that race and the suffering I saw on the runners' faces, made everything in *my* life seem easier. And I started to see the parallels between this loopy endurance race and the small businesses that were scratching out a living in my Howard Beach neighborhood. There, the daily hustle began at 4 AM. You could smell the bagels being buttered and hear the hum of delivery trucks' diesel engines as Howard Beach woke up and went to work. I was inspired by the work ethic I witnessed every day in my neighborhood and I recognized the same in those crazy transcendence runners.

In the 90s, after building a few businesses and making some money, the fire in my belly was going out. I was getting fat, feeling lousy, and losing my edge. This wasn't how I wanted to live my life. I remembered when my mom introduced me to the transcendence race and how it had such an influence on my life back then. I needed some transcendence in my own life. I started doing Bikram Yoga and running up and down stadium stairs in the lung-searing heat of summer. I loved the suffering during workouts and the feeling of exhaustion after giving my all in a race. I started signing up for all kinds of races. I was not quite ready for 3,100 miles. Physically, I had some work to do. But my resolve and resilience were strong, thanks to 10+ years of busting hump as a small business owner.

Quickly, I found myself searching for more and more competitions, all kinds of events; the longer, the harder, and the less likely it was for me to finish the race, the more I wanted in. I consumed races much like others consumed coffee. In competing around the world, I continued to recognize the similarities between extreme endurance racing, business, and life.

By 2000, I was addicted to entrepreneurial ventures and endurance racing. These were my two passions and I wanted to combine my passion for both. I purchased Peak.com and launched our first race in the British Virgin Islands. That race was 350 miles of biking, running, and kayaking, with some insane challenges thrown in between for fun. It was a terrific concept, but, like all startups, Peak faced immense, unexpected challenges immediately. Just a few months before the event, the Sept 11th attacks occurred, and we lost all of our sponsors. I was quickly $500,000 in the hole, but I would do it again tomorrow. I wouldn't change anything because I learned so much from that experience of extreme adversity. I use what I learned then every day of my life.

Fast forward 10 years and I found myself married with four kids. My life had completely changed; and I decided to retire on a farm in Vermont. But all the while, the one constant was adventure racing. I continued to race and also challenge people by putting on races that forced them to recognize their human potential. Every time I held another race, I lost some more money, but I just LOVED seeing people crush their perceived limitations. That's what it was all about. I had found my True North. I wanted to rip people off their couches and transform their lives, as mine had been transformed.

Enter the Death Race.

The goal was simple: Crush people. Absolutely crush them. Push them so far beyond their limits that they finally meet their real selves. When I think back, I remember questioning whether or not it was possible to create a sporting event that mimicked both life's challenges and the hardships of running a business. Could I manufacture situations where everything that could go wrong would go wrong, just as it is in business? I wanted to create the ultimate test of will that forced people to suffer and overcome the most grueling of obstacles. I wanted to manufacture a living hell, a race that would go on for as long as I wanted it to go on, no matter how painful or psychologically diabolical.

Ironically, the Death Race is all about life ... and growth. You only truly live when you face excruciatingly difficult challenges. You only grow when you get far out of your comfort zone. Whether you're a tree or a human being, it's when you extend yourself outside that place of ease and comfort that you begin to grow new shoots and new roots. We know this, right? That's why it's so important to face your fears and find the courage to stretch yourself like a rubber band and discover how far you can go before breaking. And if you do break, remember, there's a lot you can learn from failure.

Think about failure like this: When they test materials at a factory, whether it's steel or fabric, it doesn't matter the type—the purpose is to find the breaking point. When the material fails, the manufacturer learns something that he or she can use to make the product better, stronger, more resilient. You do the same in a Death Race. It's manufactured adversity. It's a stress-testing laboratory, a proving ground that builds your confidence in your abilities by changing your frame of reference. A Death Race is transforming. Halfway through, you're already a different person. You'll no longer waste time complaining about the silly stuff that used to bother you. Everything is much easier by comparison. You can overcome anything. And at the finish line you realize, "Holy shit! I'm a lot stronger and a lot tougher than I thought I was."

That's a powerful revelation, and it's why we need to practice facing adversity regularly. God forbid somebody gets sick, a family member dies, you get fired, or you get divorced. Shit happens. But the more proficient you are at facing these terrible adversities, the better prepared you will be for whatever life throws at you.

The only way you can gain this kind of wisdom and skill is by actually immersing yourself in it. You can't read a book or listen to a podcast and get the same knowledge. You have to earn it by suffering.

But it's suffering for a purpose. You feel the pain and work through it to gain the growth. You push through a barrier, an obstacle, and you take a mental note about how you did it, and then you go out and you repeat that. Sometimes, you fail to overcome the obstacle, you crack, you break, but you make a mental note, you gain more wisdom, and with that knowledge, you will find you can go a little further next time.

That's the pure beauty of an event as gut-wrenchingly difficult as the Death Race: It's transformative. It's transcendent. It teaches you that real growth is rewarded in buckets, physically and mentally, when you dig deeper.

When you grasp that truth, you'll believe that there's no obstacle in life that you cannot overcome..

PROLOGUE

BEFORE DEATH

After the Death Race, everything changed. After the Death Race, nothing phased me. After the Death Race, I became more stoic, immovable, and unbreakable. When I think back on it, the way I remember feeling post Death Race is much like how I imagine Edward Norton's character felt in the movie Fight Club after his first few fights. Norton is sitting in his office and he is dabbing blood off his lip when he says this line that resonates so deeply within, "After fighting, everything else in your life got the volume turned down...you could deal with anything."

The Death Race offered enlightenment similar to that which Edward Norton achieved through fighting; and since then the volume has been turned down. Way down.

After pushing myself to such extremes and subjecting myself to one of the toughest endurance events the world has to offer, I walked away a changed man. I left Vermont multiple times, each with a new outlook on life.

You know, it's funny how voluntarily paying large sums of money to chop wood, build a stone staircase, and trek countless miles – all while being told over and over how you should quit and that you could never finish this race – can change you at your very core. I could never have imagined how transformational a single encounter could be until I dove head first into the experience that would shape who I am today.

No matter how many times I was told I should quit, I somehow managed to find the courage, power, and wisdom to prove the race directors wrong, on more than one occasion. Despite all the odds, I walked away from the event known as the Death Race, with a new lease on life and, of course, with that plastic skull in hand.

The very thing that signified all the pain and glory I went through wasn't some fancy medal or a beautiful plaque; no, this was the Death Race. This was an event meant to give you a whole new frame of reference for life, one that goes beyond materialistic wants and needs. To best represent this minimalist ideal was a plastic skull that you could find on the shelf at any dollar store in middle-of-nowhere-America. And it was all the reward I would ever need. This simple skull represented much more than a token prize. It represented all the suffering required to claim the title "Death Race Finisher."

In the pages that follow is a story of a race borne out of the curiosity of two adventure-race endurance junkies who wanted nothing more than to see how far humans could go. The Death Race was a new kind of event that tested just how courageous a person is and just how powerful they can become. This "Death" Race was designed to not only test the mental and physical grit of an individual through extreme means, but also to break a person down before giving them the chance to build themselves back up again. Oftentimes, through the trials and tribulations, athletes would walk away from the event having uncovered a heightened state of being.

Whether Joe DeSena and Andy Weinberg knew it when they first started developing this race or not, that is just what they did – changed the perspective a competitor has on a particular event and themselves. In the beginning, the Death Race wasn't even its own race. It was a particular "Death Division" of the Peak Ultra Marathon that soon spun-off into its private, independent event that managed to draw the attention of over 300 endurance athletes from around the globe in just a few years. Competitors travelled to the small mountain town of Pittsfield, Vermont to gather and attempt to survive Death.

In the past two to three decades, humans have devolved into desk jockeys and couch potatoes, and in doing so, we have lost our innate ability to be primal beings capable of surviving without modern luxuries. From some perspectives, The Death Race became a social experiment that challenged people to reach the next level of human potential. The Death Race would inadvertently become a test of how capable an individual was at overcoming adversity and surviving extreme situations. And that is exactly why I had to do it. I had to find out what I was made of...that's all there was to it.

Up until this point of my life, nothing really tested my limits, nothing ever pushed me over the edge, not in the manner in which I sought most – to be pushed beyond my mental, physical, and emotional limits. As an athlete since birth, competition defined every stage of my life thus far. In gymnastics I competed at the high school and national level, and in college as a nationally ranked cheerleader. Even academically, I completed college in four years and graduate school in 18 months all while working full time. No matter what the environment was, however, nothing ever came close to "breaking" me.

Everything, for the most part, came relatively easy. School, athletics, work, all of it. But life, life is not easy. It's not supposed to be. I knew this and I wanted to see what existed out there in the world that not only could, but hopefully would break me. I needed to find out so I could ultimately prepare. Self-improvement and a growth mindset were instilled in me at a young age. In my family, we were always taught that it was within our control to continually improve our health, mind, body, and spirit. We were taught how to use these tools to create a happy life - through discipline, perseverance and a relentless pursuit toward our goals.

My personal life journey has blessed me with many talents. But if there is one thing I have learned these past 30 years, it is that talent only gets you so far and that those who work hard, typically go further than those who try to skate by on talent alone. I was blessed with plenty of natural ability, but through years of discipline practicing sports activities, I also developed an immense amount of tenacity. From my experience as an athlete, I learned what it takes to be a top achiever. I learned that putting in the hours is what it takes to come out the other side, harder, better, faster, stronger.

Preparing for the Death Race was no small feat, my experience was riddled with trials and tribulations that would force me to dig deep, but this isn't the story of my preparation, it is the story of my three years going head-to-head and toe-to-toe with Death and where it all began.

YEAR 1

COURAGE

"Life shrinks or expands in proportion to one's courage"

~Anaïs Nin

CHAPTER 1

DESTINATION: DEATH RACE, VERMONT

"The best way to make your dreams come true is to wake up."
~ Paul Valery

June 13, 2012

—

Six months, two cortisone shots and an ongoing prescription of Norco (prescription strength acetaminophen and hydrocodone) later and just like that, it was Wednesday evening. T-minus two days until the last day of my old life.

Before I hit the pillow for the evening, I already had all of my bags fully packed and ready to go. Being able to pack efficiently and quickly is something I pride myself on when traveling. For nearly all of my adventures, I can pack quite quickly without missing a thing.

This time was different. This time, the nerves of this impending race had me scrambling around the house, frantically trying to make sure there was nothing of importance hiding behind a shelf or stuffed deep in the back of a drawer. I couldn't forget anything essential.

Meanwhile, the rest of the house was fast asleep, except my father who was half awake and insisted I get some rest. I dedicated myself to one more review of my checklist. Finally, around 1:00 am my body lay still on my ultra-comfortable, king-size, memory foam mattress – the last time I would be this content until after the Death Race. And I would only get three hours to enjoy it.

Cue the iPhone alarm jingle. It was 4:15 am and I jumped to attention and let the morning kick me in the teeth. I made a quick dash to the shower. I decided to make it a comfortable one so I cranked it up to a pleasant temperature and took a moment to enjoy the delight of the nice warm shower. Time was fleeting, so I showered quickly, toweled off, dressed for the journey and gathered all my bags to put in the car. Thankfully, one of my best supporters, my mother, was willing to wake up early and drive me to the airport to wish me luck on my adventure.

After a few delays and a layover, I finally arrived at Manchester International Airport, where my friend, Mark Webb, picked me up.

It was easy to identify Mark's vehicle because he was prominent in the rucking (carrying a weighted pack for fun) community and he had a personalized GORUCK license plate on his Land Rover. He arrived just minutes after I pulled my large Eberlestock Gunslinger II pack out of baggage claim. The baggage carriers were kind enough to place my bag in large contractor bag - apparently they did not want my ax falling out.

Not knowing what to eat during an event of this length along with the requirement to carry as much food on your person as is necessary to survive a week in the woods can become expensive quickly. Mark and I made a stop at the grocery store where we each purchased four gallons of water along with bottles of Gatorade, Vitamin Water, and perhaps most importantly, a bottle of Deep Woods bug spray. With the shopping complete, we drove to Vermont to get some rest and relaxation. Mark was smart and got himself a quiet hotel to spend the night while I decided to find a free couch to sleep on at our mutual friend, Todd Sedlak's house.

As it turned out, Todd wasn't there yet and he would not arrive until the morning, cutting it really close to the race start time. Another racer, by the name of Leyla, had the same idea I did and would also be staying at Todd's. She arrived shortly after I did, prior to this we had only met through a Facebook group, now we would be finding dinner together. After fueling ourselves with some delicious carb-y pizza we went back to Todd's house to get our final rest. The next day the two of us, along with some two-hundred and fifty other individuals would take on a race that marketed itself with the web domain, www.youmaydie.com. This one last sleep was more crucial than I could have ever imagined.

On Friday morning, I woke up anxious around 5:30 am. Though I was full of angst, I was able to set that aside for a moment while I enjoyed one of the most vibrant and beautiful sunrises I had seen in my twenty-five years on this planet. Vibrant shades of orange, pink and blue filled the sky. Unfortunately, I was too tired to have the notion to take any pictures. I did snap a few photos after I was more awake to capture the remoteness of the location. With just enough time to rest, I closed my eyes and the next thing I knew it was 8:00 am. Time to get up!

I showered one last time before I would inevitably spend the next two days in my own filth. Twenty minutes later, we were ready to hit the road for a 40-minute drive from Todd's home to Pittsfield – where the Death Race festivities would begin at 10:00am. At that time, a special "HINTS" briefing would take place outside the Original General Store, at least that was the message going around. When I woke up, I found another Death Racer, Yitzy, had arrived while I was fast asleep. Leyla and I asked Yitzy if he would like to join us in attending the briefing. He participated in this race the year prior and was of the opinion that this hints briefing was most likely an unnecessary gathering designed to psych people out. He opted to stay behind.

Leyla and I took off and when we arrived the place was already a buzz. I went inside and grabbed myself a quick bite to eat, a delicious, locally-sourced, ham sandwich. I finished eating outside while the race directors Andy and Joe gathered all the

Death Racers, support crews, and whomever else was there to listen. Since I stayed separately from Mark, I only had my clothes and every day pack on my persons, all my race gear and food supplies were still in Mark's vehicle. I didn't let fear get the best of me, I was certain we still had plenty of time before the race would begin. This was merely an early morning briefing after all. It was the calm before the storm, and I was hopeful there would be some insight provided at this early briefing.

CHAPTER 2

THE BEGINNING

"Don't be intimidated by what you don't know. That can be your greatest strength and ensure that you do things differently from everyone else." ~ Sara Blakely

The "Hints" briefing was shorter than I had expected. Once I realized the information was lackluster, I started to maneuver myself away from the crowd. One thing the organizers did tell us (that I actually believed) was that we should wear shorts that night. I learned quickly that anything about the Death Race, especially at this particular incarnation – the **Year of Betrayal** – was that the truth remained elusive.

Anything and everything could be a betrayal. Joe and Andy could be telling the truth or lying. The volunteer staff could be helping or sabotaging your race – there was no way to know. The **Year of Betrayal** was a fitting moniker indeed.

As I left the briefing, I had not figured out Joe and Andy's game yet. I was not sure how to tell if they were steering us in the right direction or betraying us. Were they lying through their teeth or telling me solid advice for the events to come? I asked that question during every interaction I had at the race. The theme of betrayal put my guard on high alert. It took a lot of courage just to sign up for this race. It took even more to show up. And it would require even more courage to trust anyone during the event.

After the briefing, we were instructed to take a look at some pieces of paper with illustrations of what was considered to be "useful" hints. Instead of posting these hint sheets somewhere everyone can see them, the organizers placed them on the ground where a bunch of Death Racers quickly huddled around them obstructing everyone else's view. At the time, the hints seemed useless, but I thought to snap a few photos on my iPhone for future reference. It might seem silly, but yes, I brought my iPhone along for the entirety of the Death Race. I kept the phone protected in a small Pelican case, I figured I could use my phone to take notes and photos when (and if) the opportunity presented itself.

For the time being, these seemingly random images were imprinted in my mind. I could vividly recall them without looking. Oftentimes, I can have a photographic memory of things, and with the importance the race directors imposed upon us, my excited mind took in every single minor detail. These images were locked in my mind. One 8.5" x 11" sheet of paper there is a coloring book image of a crawling baby and with a sharpie its eyes are crossed out, and the word NO is written in all caps and double underlined. Another sheet is beside it with the words "VOMIT IS OK" centered, bold, and in all caps. While another three sheets lay side-by-side all depicting the same scene. The scene looked like it might be taken from a Bible coloring book and it appeared to be a picture of Jesus with one of his disciples placing a hand on his shoulder, both men were standing in front of six soldiers. On the far left sheet each soldier was labeled with a number one through six written above their heads, on the middle sheet there is a circle drawn around the disciple's hand on Jesus's shoulder and an arrow is drawn to point toward the circle, the number three is written in sharpie below Jesus and the number four below the disciple. On the far right the left foot of who I presume was Jesus is circled, there is a capital 'A' written on the center of the disciple, and the most aggressive looking soldier has a circle drawn around his head. All of these images, including the bear with the inner tube around his waist, seemed meaningless. Sure they probably in some way hinted at what was to come, but from my perspective, it seemed like these "hints" were merely meant to confuse and intimidate. Only time would reveal their true meaning.

Impatient and unsure what to do until the event began, I called Mark. When I found out he was still about 20 minutes away, I took the opportunity to wait inside the General Store and calm my nerves - I did not know when I would have the chance to "relax" again.

Upon Mark's arrival at the store, we organized our belongings in his car and we made our way back down to the farm to unload our food, extra clothing and supplies at the racers' tents.

We finished up shortly after, but not before two friends, Mies and Chris showed up with a garbage bag filled with human hair. It was one of the more perplexing gear list items, but we had to get everything on the list. It just so happens that, Mies is a hair stylist and she was kind enough to grab a nice stash for all of us before leaving the salon. We would not discover the purpose of the human hair until the end of the race and I would owe a great deal to Mies and Chris for saving the day by supplying our crew with the bags of human hair that we so desperately needed. Quickly, I grabbed my small amount and threw it in a Ziploc and also bagged some for Todd who was still not anywhere close to arriving.

With our bags of hair secured, Mark and I moved his car down the road to a parking spot over at Amee Farm and made our way toward the mountain that we had to climb. On the way up the gravel road, we hopped in a pickup truck with a fellow racer by the name of Eric, and his support crew. We shared some laughs about our impending "doom" as we drove as far up Tweed River Drive as we could before we had to get out for the final ascent up "Joe's" Mountain. The route where you take Tweed River Drive from Riverside Farm to the top of the mountain is approximately three miles and 1,000 feet of elevation gain. By catching a ride a quarter of a mile into our journey, we were able to skip about two to two and a half miles and about 600 to 700 feet of climbing.

We drove until the road turned to gravel, and we could see

things looked a bit sketchy with everyone gathering here. There, outside the quiet town of Pittsfield, we began the first of what would be many hikes up the mountainsides of Vermont with all of our gear in tow.

As far as gear is concerned, a racer's equipment is crucial to survival and success in this race. Without the required materials and tools, finishing is highly unlikely. An essential participatory requirement was that we were to always carry a handwritten list of all of the items that we planned to have with us during the race. At any time during the event, the event organizers could request a bag inspection and should an item not be present, we would get our first warning and a penalty. The second offense meant disqualification.

As we hiked away from the pickup truck and around a switchback that continued to climb further up the mountain, we noticed other vehicles had been able to navigate further up the mountain. Fortunately for us, a racer by the name of Rod had family on their way down, they kindly scooped us up and drove our small crew closer to our final destination for the official weigh-in.

After we were dropped off by Rod's family, we finally we hit the trail and hiked our way to the top of the mountain. Once there, we were met with a long line we had to wait in. The excitement of when the race would start left me anxious with anticipation. While we waited, a few kids with blindingly bright, fluorescent yellow Death Race volunteer shirts were walking around with cups of rabbit food.

The youngsters were tasked with handing out a minimum of two pieces to each racer and told us that we were to keep hold of the rabbit food until the end of the race. Otherwise, we would face a penalty. In some moment of frustration, a racer cursed aloud near the young ones, leading to a warning that the next person to swear would get given as many burpees as the children found amusing. I found it best to stay silent, for the most part, and observe.

Our group was held back from moving forward in the line a few times since those who were monitoring the whole ordeal were giving VIP treatment to previous Death Racers and to females, allowing them to jump to the front of the line.

It turned out that Winter Death Racers finishers were not included in this VIP treatment as Mark and Eric pleaded their case, but were told that a Winter Death Race finish didn't count. What a blow to the ego. I feared the Winter Death Race, the awful cold that participants are subjected to is just unbearable.

As I walked up to the weigh-in station, I was instructed to provide the volunteers with my name and asked to step on the scale with my ruck and all of my gear. I came in at 197-lbs.

To provide some context, before training for the Death Race, I typically weighed anywhere from 160-165-lbs. As the Death Race approached, I found myself averaging anywhere from 152-158-lbs. The week leading up to the race I did not exercise, lift, or run in order to avoid injuring myself before the biggest race of my life. I also tried to eat as much food and carbohydrates as possible to pack on some weight that I was certain I would quickly burn off over the course of the weekend.

It was a priority in my mind that I did not finish the race weighing anything less than 150-lbs. The thought of my weight being so low for my frame was disconcerting. I had not weighed under 155-lbs since high school. Now, I'm not sure how accurate the scale at the weigh-in was (it looked old) but at home, my pack weighed in around 35-lbs total. Some quick math would suggest that my body weight at weigh-in was close to 162-lbs; based on my average weight, it was safe to assume the scale was off anywhere from 4-8-lbs. In the grand scheme of things, it was close enough.

Once our group was all weighed in, we made our way back down to the truck. From there, we took a ride back down to Riverside Farm to finish our race registration. Inside we were asked repeatedly by volunteers if we were sure we wanted to race or if we wanted to quit. Looking back, I apologize to all the volunteers for being a bit haughty with all my snide laughs at their questions – I figure they knew it was all in good fun.

As soon as we completed registration we were given a Peak Races t-shirt, a hat, and our bib number. I was bib number 559. Upon leaving the registration cabin, we were directed to go outside and speak with "the guy in the hat" for our first task/challenge. The three of us walked up to "the guy in the hat" and waited for him to begin his instructions.

Our mission was simple: we had to complete if we wanted to compete. The first task was to sew the bib number we were just given to the required black top we had to wear. It was a good thing I packed my needle and thread when I first received the gear list – it seemed like an odd gear list item – but as I had just discovered, it was required.

Since we had some time until the scheduled race start, our group headed over to the Original General Store to complete this task. Using a strip of cloth from a large scarf of Eric's, we each cut off our own section to use. We cut our piece up into the shape of our bib numbers and then we sewed the cloth numbers on while enjoying our last real meal. As the clock hands approached six, we succumbed to the fact that it was time to head over to Amee Farm. With our bib numbers sewn on, we waited to see what our next task would be.

This is where the race began.

CHAPTER 3

CRAWLING UNDER HIGHWAYS, PINK SWIM CAPS, AND SLOSH PIPES

"You only live once, but if you do it right, once is enough." ~ Mae West

As we adorned our fancy new "bibs", I tried not to let the reality of not receiving the iconic Death Race bib get to me, but to be unreserved, I was upset. The simplistic design of the Death Race bib I had seen on racers from previous years were quite spiffy. The typical bib was an all white sleeveless polyester material with the words DEATH RACE in bold red Impact font along with each unique bib number in black below. How could I not want one? I wasn't desperate, but I really wanted one and to my momentary sadness, that was not happening at the 2012 **Year of Betrayal**.

Focused and ready for our first task, I reported to this boisterous and wildly animated character by the name of Don. He was constantly making these large gestures with his arms and his body and he was quite vocal about how none of us would finish the race. With such a loud mouth I started referring to him as "Sergeant Screamer", it seemed fitting. When we reported to him, we were to show him our newly stitched bibs. If he approved of the size of the handmade bib numbers, he would check our name off and mark this task as complete. At least that is what I assumed. I do not recall seeing a list, but you would think the race organizers would keep track of this sort of thing, right?

When Mark, Eric, and I approached Sergeant Screamer we were each told that our bib numbers were not the required four inches in height and were informed that we would receive our penalty at a later time. For the first time, this is where the theme – the **Year of Betrayal** – resonated in my mind. Not one of us recalled an instruction indicating a four inch height requirement for our bib numbers, but here we were being told that we would be penalized later for not doing something that, as far as we were concerned, was never instructed.

Regardless of whether we were right or wrong, we accepted the decision and carried on our way. One by one, we began our crawl through a somewhat narrow and dark culvert that tunneled under Route 100, which is the main road running through the town of Pittsfield. This culvert was tight, very long, and absolutely pitch black. The only useful senses were our ability to touch and to hear as we felt and listened to each other move through the dark space.

Personally, I have never been one to get claustrophobic, but a little over halfway through this crawl that feeling changed. As I followed behind Mark, I occasionally had to stop because my hand would grab onto his shoe instead of touching the metal floor of the pipe. With each step further into the darkness, my heart started to race. I felt the anxiety beginning to brew within my ribcage. I closed my eyes...took a deep breath, calmed my mind and exhaled slowly. At this moment, I reassured myself, "You are going to be fine, just a little further and you will see the light and soon after you will be back outside."

Immediately after my meditative moment, I heard someone ahead of both Mark and I yell back that they could see the light.

Halle-fuckin-lujah!

I exhaled a sigh of relief, I knew there was no way this tunnel could go on forever. As we neared the end of the tunnel, I could see that Mark had lifted himself ever so slightly onto his toes and used his hands to raise the rest of his body off the ground.

Apparently, there were few jagged parts up ahead. It quickly made sense why he had stopped crawling like a baby and I quickly followed suit.

After emerging from the tunnel, we ran back across the street when it was all clear. Our next directive was to grab another item from our gear list. This time, it was the pink swim cap and our life jackets. All signs pointed to a dip in the water so I strapped myself into a slightly oversized life jacket I borrowed from my parents' neighbors and I opened the packaging to the sexy pink swim cap in preparation for a quick splash in the pond.

Next, we made our way back across the street near where we had emerged from the culvert. We were told we had to swim out to the yellow buoy, go around it, and then swim back. Simple enough. To make things more fun and entertaining, the race staff and volunteers were instructed to tell us that the pond was filled with diseases and such, including E.coli.

Yay!

To this day I don't know whether or not that was a scare tactic or the cold hard truth. That pond water was absolutely vile.

After the swim, we headed back across Route 100 yet again to receive the next task. For many, the fabled wood-chopping that became a staple of the Peak Death Race would be the next task. For me, it was time to cross that street again to re-stack some of the wood stockpiles where the rest of the wood being chopped would eventually end up. It was tricky to reorganize this pile thanks to a poorly-parked SUV directly in front of the wood pile.

Before I ran across the street, I finally saw Todd! I honestly started to wonder if he was going to make it in time, plus, I wanted desperately to rid myself of the additional off-putting bag of human hair. As soon as I saw him, I made a quick detour and handed the bag over to him.

At first, the wood stacking segment was simply a bunch of racers grabbing wood, running around the SUV, laying it down and running back for more. Once enough of us had made our way over to the wood stacking area, we quickly switched tactics and utilized the most apparent form of teamwork for this task — we formed an assembly line. I was at the front of the stockpile; therefore, I became one of the participants that became responsible for the separation of useful firewood and scraps that were better-suited for the fire pits throughout the weekend.

Our group had to remove a few stacks of wood that were piled over six feet high, and stacked three layers deep. As a group, we merely passed all of the wood that was poorly stacked back to be held until we had enough removed to fix the trouble areas that were affecting the quality of the stacks' appearance. Once that trouble spot was adjusted we began to restock and align everything to make it perfectly presentable for anyone wanting to grab some wood to heat the lodge that coming winter.

As our pile of wood dwindled down, we were told that we were "running out of time" according to a volunteer named Connor. He was monitoring our progress and made suggestions as to what would be considered an "acceptable" stack. A handful of racers were selected to head back across the road to Amee Farm while a few of us were left behind to finish.

It did not take long for me to learn that, in the Death Race, being at the front or back of anything can have a negative impact on how your personal race will go. In later years, I had learned from my observations that it was best to position yourself somewhere in the middle of the pack. Since this was my first engagement with the Death Race, and things were just getting started, I found myself where I normally wanted to be in any race, or anything I have ever participated in, somewhere in the front of the pack. Thanks to my foolhardiness, I found myself with a few others accumulating extra work and we were forced to stack the remainder of the pile.

After quickly finishing the stacking task, I went and grabbed my pack from behind the small shed. Because it was the **Year of Betrayal**, I found myself continually thinking ahead as to how I could be betrayed and having my pack stolen seemed like one of the most appropriate betrayals.

Once I grabbed my pack, I ran back to Amee Farm to find out that the race staff and volunteers were collecting all critical items that no Death Racer would leave behind, primarily State IDs or Driver's Licenses, car keys, or anything relatively important that a person would not leave behind when it was time to go home. This was meant to ensure a level of safety, it was a simple measure to keep track of the racers and easily identify anyone who had not collected their personal belongings when it was all over. I made the mistake of leaving my wallet in my everyday backpack which was still in Mark's vehicle, that was where I also stored extra pain medicine in case I needed it after the race was over.

I saved additional medications back at the car because I only wanted to bring what was considered an appropriate dosage to take over the course of the next 50-60 hours. I brought what I figured would be enough to get me through the race and stored it in my Ziploc baggie.

Since I was not able to check in without my wallet and my ID for a few minutes I had to scramble and search around for Adam, who had Mark's keys. While I rushed around, there was a group of racers who had already checked-in and were now tasked with holding various objects above their heads including, kayaks, slosh pipes, and one monster of a tire.

A slosh pipe is large in diameter (five or six inches at least). This one was filled three-quarters of the way with water giving the water just enough space to allow it to slosh around from side to side. With every step, every movement, the water also moved. This creates quite the dynamic. Finding equilibrium is key. Teamwork is essential.

Just before a sense of panic found its way into my head, I was able to spot Adam. Together, we hustled over to Mark's car, I hastily grabbed my ID from my wallet and sprinted back to the check-in table. I proclaimed my bib number to the volunteers and dropped my ID on the table with a determined sense of purpose. I had already dared to sign-up and show up to this event, I could not let a simple mistake get in the way of this race.

After successfully averting that crisis, I quickly squirmed my way into a spot next to Mark underneath one of the slosh pipes. There were so many racers and so few objects I could barely get a full hand on the tube. The sloshing of all the water in the pipe makes for a fun balancing act, which becomes even more interesting when the pipe is long enough that it requires a ten person team to carry it. With people of varied heights, the challenge to keep the water equally distributed makes communication and shuffling around a huge necessity to ensure everyone shares the load.

We all stood there, ruck-less while holding these objects above our heads when suddenly, the race directors demanded everyone to immediately head across the street. In my mind, I was uncertain about leaving my pack behind. Since I had already made it a conscious decision to always place my bag somewhere safe, I stashed my ruck in the racers' tent for safe keeping. With betrayal on my mind, I really did not know who or what to trust, except for my instinct.

As soon as we made it across Route 100 and set down the objects near the disease-ridden pond, we were quickly reprimanded for not bringing our packs along with us at all times. I somewhat expected this to happen the moment I put my pack down – I did not trust my instinct and went with the crowd. From that point on, our packs were to be on us at all times. A mad scramble of racers charged across Route 100 as everyone ran back to the farm to find their bags and regroup again at the pond.

Upon our return, we were informed it was time to get our lifejackets on once again, it was time to take a bath and into the "E.coli-infested" pond we all went. While I did not believe that this pond was actually an E.coli-infested pond as was inferred, the water was clearly repugnant so I remained extremely cautious. While I bobbed up and down across the pond, I tightly squeezed my lips together. I only opened my mouth when it was necessary to speak a question, or command, otherwise my lips were sealed.

As we continued to float around, race directors, Joe and Andy, began providing all of the athletes with instructions about how the race would proceed. To begin, we broke up into teams and had to start the race working with our team to head out on what, unbeknownst to us, would probably go down in history as one of the most legendary hikes in the history of the Death Race.

Shortly after this briefing, a large box of ping pong balls was flung into the water, and we were all to grab one, which would determine our team number. There were 10 teams, so the ping pong balls had sharpie scribbled numbers from 1 to 10. Some, however, had various messages such as "you will fail" or "give up now" or even "disqualified" written on them. As luck would have it, I picked one of the "give up now" balls first. I quickly tossed it away and looked for another. I found number 10 and then gathered along the edges of the pond with the other racers. The sides of the pond were shallow enough that you could actually stand, so we positioned ourselves with our fellow teammates. I was surprised at how quickly we were able to get organized as usually when you try to get a bunch of people to rally together, it doesn't usually go smoothly at first.

Once everyone found the team to which they belonged, we made our way out of the pond one team-unit at a time. We were to locate our packs, gather our team, and grab one of the team-carry objects. After having been doing random tasks for hours, things were still only just getting started. It was finally time to go on our first hike. At this point, the race directors taunted us, reciting things like, "We hope you brought enough food and water because we will be gone most of the night."

Betrayal? No, this was not betrayal, not yet, the race directors were 100 percent earnest, and yet most of us did not believe them, which lead to the need for us to distribute and share food among our other competitors later on.

Myself and the rest of the team grabbed our slosh pipe and trickled in with the other teams as we made our initial ascent. The hike that would eventually lead to Bloodroot Mountain began as the sun slowly fell behind the mountains and cast a shadow over all of us.

CHAPTER 4

BLOODROOT

"Great achievement is usually born of great sacrifice, and is never the result of selfishness." ~ Napoleon Hill

It was still light out, but just barely. We were on our first challenge as a team heading up into the mountains of Vermont. We would soon be on our way toward one of the most wicked, switchback-infested, and narrow passages I have ever encountered. The passing lane would be so tight that we feared losing someone the entire evening. In fact, we genuinely worried that someone might fall off the edge of the mountainside and tumble into the void. This part of the journey took place on one of the steeper, more treacherous mountains in the range in which we were nestled, following a trail known as Bloodroot Mountain Trail. Bloodroot is over 18 miles of hell, which we would spend close to 12 hours traversing.

However, let us slow down a little and get back to the first challenge as a team.

During the initial ascent, we found ourselves adjusting to our team – and to our team weight – in many ways. After introductions with our new teammates, we moved straight into conceiving, developing, and rapidly-deploying a system that divided the burden of carrying the slosh pipe. At first, no one was aware of the importance of equally distributing the water in the slosh pipe. I offered a suggestion that we allocate the weight based on our individual heights and the grade of the ascent. By placing taller people at the back and shorter people at the front on the inclines and using the reverse for the declines, we could effectively keep the water inside the slosh pipe in some sort of equilibrium. Once the plan was in place, it made it simple to carry, and we would quickly change our setup depending on what surface we were on, be it flat, an incline or a decline.

We only required four or five people to carry the slosh pipe at a time. As we trekked along the trail, the MacGyver in each of us came out and offered up new ideas that would lead to more efficient ways to handle this massive piece of *fun and joy*. Some elements of this portion of the race are a bit hazy to remember with all the excitement and adrenaline surging through my veins, but I do remember that everything was happening rapidly with a high level of intensity and purpose.

Suddenly, someone from the race staff made a point to relay a message to everyone that whichever team arrived last to the next checkpoint would be eliminated from the race. Hearing this news, Team Ten cranked things up to eleven. Our team connected on a very basic level. We had a purpose, we had an objective, and most importantly, we had an incentive to not be last, so we sped up. We were flying past everyone! Instead of remaining in a peaceful line of groups ascending the mountain, here we were barreling ahead.

People took quick notice of the sudden shift in the urgency of our team and others and followed suit. The possibility of being disqualified this early on was maddening, and naturally, the event-wide message that the last group would be booted from the race created a less than safe experience.

Racers began to forget they were going through a mountain pass with kayaks and heavy objects. Many racers stopped taking proper precautions when trying to pass other teams because they were too concerned with their own well-being and status in the race. Those of us with slosh pipes definitely had an advantage with how little space we took up. As a group, we were still somewhat narrow, enabling us to pass with greater ease than the other teams.

As we forced our way up and down, and up and down all of the rolling ascents and descents we suddenly found ourselves at a dead end where all of the teams were directed to immediately turn around. Team Ten was somewhere in the front of the pack as we were among the first three teams to arrive. This was a very interesting way for the race directors to shake things up. All the teams that thought they were sitting in the front of the pack, were now in the back. From first to last, just-like-that. Everyone who had fallen behind suddenly had the upper hand. We could not let this slick move interfere with how we would perform. Our team, Team Ten, was comprised of a group of individuals who, on their own, possessed incredible athleticism, together, we were damn near unstoppable. It only took what felt like just a few brief minutes before we found our entire team with our slosh pipe on our shoulders, back at the front of the pack. Nothing could stop us.

Team Ten had the drive to excel. It was absolutely thrilling to be a part of such a dominant group of human beings. It had been a long time coming as the past few team events I had participated in had revealed a massive gap regarding the athletic capacity of others in comparison to myself. For me, this gap hindered my level of enjoyment. Many events left me disappointed, but the Death Race made quick work of showing me what I wanted and needed to experience in a team environment.

Team Ten and all the Death Racers were a collection of driven machines. Not only were we working very well together, but we were also kicking some ass and rockin' out. Team Ten had the oldest and youngest of the Death Race together on the team. We were a diverse group of racers that came from all over. Yet, here we all were working together as if we had known each other forever. We were one group, acting as a single unit, and simply put our squad was merely taking an order, and executing at our highest potential. Team Ten charged back to the front soon enough. It is hard to determine, specifically in the moment, and even now when looking back on everything, whether we were overexerting ourselves to hold our position, or if together we were at our best. Regardless, jointly we all felt fantastic, so why not keep the pace?

As I recall, when we reached the first of a few pit stops, we were instructed to complete any given number of burpees as directed at each stop. Of course, to keep all of us on our toes, the race directors created intentional confusion by splitting up and taking different routes. Andy took off in one direction, and Joe took another path. There was one team in front of us that followed Andy. We were tempted to follow Andy but realized we were being tricked and cut back to take Joe's route. Joe did not like that we were on to him, so he kept prodding us, "Are you sure this is the right decision?"

We refused to fall for his deceptive tactics. As a result of our ability to make a decision as a team and not fall for the deception, we were congratulated, and together we pressed onward. I am not sure what happened to the other team that broke and followed Andy's path, but there was no time to pay attention to what the other teams were doing. My focus, our focus, had to be directed wholly at our crew. Team Ten was back in first. This could be good, or this could be bad.

We arrived at the first burpee-filled rest stop. If you were not hiking, you were probably doing something else, like burpees. And since that meant we did not have to carry our packs, I considered that rest. I was overcome with happiness, for the first time since we started the hike we were allowed to relieve ourselves of wearing our packs. It was a welcome shift. Now our shoulders could rest, if only briefly.

As a group, we placed all of our packs in the middle of a circle formed by our team. At this time, we still had 21 members on Team Ten, leaving us with a decently-sized circle to form. We were instructed to begin with 100 burpees for all. As other teams joined in making their own circles, we had to continue our burpees, regardless of how many we had already completed. Arriving first had a peculiar advantage, it turned out we would be doing more burpees than we were initially instructed to perform.

Team Ten created a steady system for cranking out these burpees, for the first few rounds, we would pound out 25 at a time. Then as reality set in and we realized we were doing more than 100, we dialed it back to sets of ten burpees for each set. At the completion of each set of ten, there would be a 5-second countdown. Once we heard someone shout the number one, we all dropped to the ground and began our next set of ten burpees with the precision of synchronized swimmers. We were in-tune. The number of burpees kept increasing by a hundred every-time someone was caught standing around from the other groups. We did our best not to break our cadence.

After having completed some 300 burpees or so, there was no way of knowing how many we would be required to complete, but I expected it could reach as many as 600 or 700. Sergeant Screamer looked over at us at one point, we were right in front of the truck he stood on with his loud-ass megaphone. As he looked over, he questioned how many burpees our team had done. As one, we shouted out the collective number. He seemed dumbfounded at first. It was then that we heard one of the most uplifting comments since the race began. Sergeant Screamer actually praised our team and said everyone else should be following our example. Our goal was simple: work together and be awesome. That's it. We eventually stopped the burpees somewhere in the mid- four to five hundred range. And here I had thought our shoulders were about to get a rest. Ha.

It should come as no surprise that I would be adding more pain to the shoulders momentarily. Instead of suffering pain inflicted by my pack or hundreds of burpees, it would be another activity that would light my shoulders on fire, figuratively speaking, of course. But that is the intensity of the pain I was experiencing at the moment. In the next task, as a team, we were to lift our object: slosh pipe, kayak, or tire above our heads. Once your team had the team-weight hoisted above you and your teammate's heads, you were to pass it around your team's circle. Team Ten used this time to start rehydrating, which we had already implemented a system for previously during the burpees, as needed.

It is incredible that I can still remember chowing down on my first Mint Chocolate Chip Clif Builder's Bar during this task. I can taste it simply by thinking about it. At the time, it was revitalizing. Immediately after consuming it, my energy levels rose up, and we, of course, were caught snacking and drinking. So, naturally, we were given a second slosh pipe. This rendered us to the point where there was only a half second of rest between each teammate receiving and passing the slosh pipe. No more snacks, or water breaks. Excellent work, race directors. You stayed true to your authoritative actions in this game, but we were unaffected by it.

We needed to ration our supplies anyway so we got what we needed out of it, even if it meant a little more work for us than everyone else. The truth is, the next part of the journey would only get worse and worse as we moved deeper into the mountainside as we would soon find ourselves facing a purposefully chaotic whirlwind orchestrated by the organizers as they led us on the trek to Bloodroot Mountain Trail. As torturous as it was, it ended up being more than worth it.

After passing the objects around in a circle over our heads for a considerable amount of time, we were instructed to place them on the ground, to grab our packs, put them on, and switch items with another team. There was one item that all groups wanted desperately to avoid. You could see it in every racer's eyes, the displeasure at the thought of this object being their team's weight as it approached. The one and only, massive, round, black tractor tire.

Before we began moving, it became clear that now would be a good time to start taking my pain relievers. For the past six months, I found myself training and battling a one-inch tear in the labrum of my left shoulder. It was a shoulder joint tear that was unpleasantly thrust upon me the day after I signed up for this race and to this day it has limited some of my range of motion. A New Years Eve spent in the hospital was not what I had had in mind, but some bully of a doorman needed to let out some rage and I was the unfortunate victim. It took a few weeks for me to discover it was torn and by then, the doctor told me I couldn't make it any worse, so I decided to go all in on my training for this race, I didn't want my $500 registration fee to go to waste after all. Days before leaving for Vermont I went to see my doctor one more time. This visit was for my second cortisone shot to ensure that my shoulder would NOT be the reason I quit.

I knew that I had to continually monitor my shoulder's status and be aware that the cortisone was taking away most of the pain. I constantly reminded myself to be careful. My prescription was for Norco and it was to be taken in a dose of one-to-two tablets every three-to-four hours as needed with food. I always opted for the lesser amount and planned to adjust accordingly. The only thing I had to worry about was if they ever did not allow us to eat, that would wreak havoc on my stomach, one of the many things that I worried about.

For the next 24 hours or so I would stick to taking one tablet every three-and-a-half to four hours. I stored a bottle back in Mark's SUV and had brought somewhere around 10 tablets with me for the race. I figured that would be enough to get me through the race. A misjudgment that would later force me to ask the crew member's of other racers for help.

Onward and out, we began the trek through Bloodroot Mountain Trail. In all the madness of the shuffle to grab an item, I'm not quite sure how our team was so unfortunate to wind up with the worst item available, but there we were forced to face the most obnoxiously large tire I had ever handled.

As it turned out, all of the successful strategies we utilized for carrying the slosh pipe were rendered useless now that we had this massive tire to navigate through a single track trail. Just before entering Bloodroot Mountain Trail, the race directors notified the group that anyone who was unable to complete 18 miles of hiking through the night should pack their bags and head back to Riverside Farm now.

At the time, I did not know if anyone actually took the offer to quit, though later I discovered there were quite a few who chose to use this as their exit from the race. Everyone has their own reason, but for me, things were just getting started, and quitting was not something I ever wanted to do. If I were pulled medically that would be one thing, or if a permanent injury was a factor, but to just voluntarily quit, that is not how you succeed at life and that was not in the cards for me. I would NOT quit.

Up until now, this event felt very reminiscent of the Spartan Race Hurricane Heat: everyone was placed in a team, camaraderie was an essential element of success, and we had an entire evening to get to know each other while hauling an enormous tire through a dangerous pass. OK, so dragging a massive tire through the most perilous pass you've ever been on may not be the same kind of thing you would encounter at a Hurricane Heat, but honestly, what more could anyone wish for? What we were doing was pretty damn incredible, no matter how dumb it may seem from the outside.

With the tire, we put forth a respectable effort to proceed with carrying the tire as we were expected – overhead. But reality soon slapped us for wasting our energy. We could not keep up, the pass was far too narrow, and, despite the url that had initially drawn me in, we didn't actually want to die. As we fell increasingly behind, our team would eventually resort to rolling the tire. We tried everything from carrying it with ropes, using our axes as handles, and even hoisting it on four or five teammates' shoulders at a time.

We even took posts and rope to try and push and pull the tire along as it rolled.

Many of these strategies worked initially, mainly when we were on the fire roads where the path was wide enough for four people carrying a tire. However, as the ascent continued, they were rendered useless as the trail narrowed the further we traveled. It would not be long before we were stopped to help a team that, surprisingly, was further behind than us.

I was stunned when we made that discovery. As it turned out, their teammate blew out his knee and we helped take on the added burden of supporting him. We continued to struggle with our own issues with the tire but nevertheless, we still trudged onward and made our way toward the next checkpoint where more burpees await. No matter the challenge we faced, we had no choice but to carry-on, so carry-on we did.

CHAPTER 5

THE TRIBULATIONS OF TEAM TIRE

"Muddy water is best cleared by leaving it alone." - Alan Watts

Over the course of six to eight hours, our team, Team Ten, rocked out. Our team conquered every challenge thrown our way. That good fortune would eventually come to an end as the difficulty of navigating this massive tire through a single track trail would start to shine a spotlight on those who were too weak or perhaps too lazy to contribute to the cause of getting the tire to our destination – wherever that may be.

The troubles that damn tire caused us took the Death Race to an all new level for everyone. All of the other teams were miles ahead of us. While we were stuck negotiating the treacherous single track trails, the rest of the racers were subjected to burpees for a long time before being allowed some rest while they waited for our team to catch up. The fact is, we never did catch up. That tire relentlessly tried to crush our souls, our collective and individual spirit.

After the other racers ahead of us were allowed their short rest, they made their way toward the Chittenden Reservoir with their kayaks and slosh-pipes. Once those teams reached the reservoir, they were all relieved of carrying their objects. They were then subjected to a swim in the reservoir before making the trek back to Riverside Farm. While all of the other teams kept progressing through the race, our team continued to traverse across the dangerous Bloodroot Mountain Trail with that blasted tire.

What I started to realize, as we moved on, was the imbalance in the distribution of time people spent with that unforgiving tire. You see, we were unable to ever have more than five people on the tire at a time. And, as Bloodroot Mountain Trail narrowed to being only single track trails, we could manage to have two to three people on the tire. The third person would usually be on the outer part of the trail because there was nowhere to fit on the inside. The chances of someone falling off and sliding down the side of the mountain were incredibly high. I am still in a state of bewilderment as to how we beat those odds and survived without injury.

The most significant pain point for Team Ten was the over-ambitious nature of half the team while the other half coasted and focused on conserving their energy. Those of us that were gung-ho about keeping the tire moving at the fastest safe pace possible would get frustrated and step up, sometimes too soon to give others a chance to move up. Most of us did not want the momentum to come to a stop. Multiple times we had to operate under what was similar to an Indian Run. Three people would drop all the way to the back, and the next batch moved forward. I tended to only fall back three-quarters of the way to the rear of the pack; I did not feel comfortable being all the way behind my team. For whatever reason, when I am at the back, I will let myself slow down even more. However, when there are people behind me and I am "chased" – I keep a more consistent pace.

Around this time, I took my second dose of painkillers. We had already gone through multiple burpee stops, and fallen way behind the rest of the pack. Everything we did was in darkness until the next morning.

I found out I wasn't alone in experiencing pain. One of my teammates was also experiencing an immense amount of pain, so I hooked her up with some aspirin. When she expressed she was still in pain hours later, I reluctantly shared some of my stronger pain medicine. Later, we would find out that she was competing on a fractured heel. Giving her that medication would help her last a little longer, and for me, would mean I would be short some pills at a time when I would need them most.

Of course, I do not regret sharing my medicine with her if it could help her make it that much farther and survive these treacherous switchbacks, climbs, and descents. This segment of the race was all about teamwork and I was more than happy to help my fellow racers in any way I could. Even though it is a race where there are both team and individual segments, the camaraderie never dissipated the entire race. We were all in the thick of it, together. We were fighting; fighting to survive all the mental and physical objectives the race directors devised.

When we had reached what we'll call the halfway point, our leaders, Joe and Andy, made an announcement. If you were not able to continue, now was the time to turn back. They had an ATV on its way up to pick up the person with the knee injury and they would be leaving anyone who did not have it in them to carry on.

Here was the last time we would see anyone other than our immediate teammates for many, many hours. We had to continue to navigate with the tire all throughout the night. I remember as the night went on some tensions would build but, thankfully, those tensions quickly subsided.

The longer it took us to navigate with the tire, the more we became concerned with dehydration. Many of us were conserving every last drop of water. For the most part, I felt like I was doing an excellent job of managing my water consumption so toward the end of this trail from Hell I shared my water with those who ran dry many hours prior. Having a minimum of a three-liter bladder is a must when you don't know how long you will be away from a water source; that little extra weight is totally worth it.

Not only were we dehydrated but most of us were also low on food. We had gone through our baggies of trail mix, slurped down our remaining gel packs, and chomped away at the last of our energy and protein bars. We all shared food, but even so, our rations grew scarce.

As the sun began to rise, we neared the end of Bloodroot Mountain Trail. I remember the breath of life that made its way back into us as those rays of light made their way over the mountains and shone through the trees. It was a marvelous sight to take in, but only for a moment as our focus had to remain on that godforsaken tire. Those fleeting moments of beauty that surrounded us came and went in an instant; then it was back to navigating the tight pass. After a few more ascents and descents, we pushed the tire over roots and squeezed our way between trees while the dead leaves crunched beneath our feet, finally making it to a clearing where we saw Joe waiting for us.

Joe had been waiting for us all night next to a smoldering fire. At first, I thought he was tied up when I saw him sitting on the ground, "Betrayal?" I thought. Quickly, I realized my eyes were playing tricks on me; it turned out he had wrapped himself in a black garbage bag. Even Joe DeSena needs to stay warm through the wee hours of the night.

Upon our arrival, we were informed that we had fallen approximately six hours behind the rest of the racers. Joe presented us with two options. Option A involved us heading out to the Chittenden Reservoir as a group to try to catch up on what we missed out on so far. Option B was to wait for the rest of the teams to come back, with no knowledge of how long that might take. Instead of letting our body's muscles seize up, we opted to keep moving forward. There was some temptation to hang out, but ultimately we knew it was best to push forward.

Joe suggested that we leave the tire there for the time being, but made it clear that we would be back for it. We all headed out towards this next checkpoint together, this is where you could see who was struggling. Some people took off and others hung back moving slowly. The rest fell somewhere in the middle and I was somewhere in that middle. I started off in the front but then a fellow racer, Damien, who managed to wear that damn pink bathing cap for the entire race, took off on the run with Joe.

At that moment, many of us on Team Ten began to suspect Damien of being a mole. He wasn't, but for a period we were all questioning this decision of his to take off without any of us. Did he know something? Was this on purpose? Is he going to get us penalized? We eventually lost sight of Joe and Damien, and then came to a turn where we were uncertain which direction they went.

I tried using my phone to pull up a map, but the effort was futile, service was nonexistent. There was just enough service available that a few text messages were able to make it through when I took my phone out of airplane mode. I received a few texts from my friend Jennifer who I had met previously at other events. She was coming up to help crew me throughout the race. Her message informed me that she was still en route to Pittsfield at that time. As thankful as I was that she was coming to support me, I would not see her until Sunday morning.

After a few minutes of trying to figure out if we should continue on, we decided to head down the road but quickly hesitated. Everyone started to think that we should go back to where we had dropped the tire. There we found ourselves once again, undecided on how to proceed as a team. Just as we started heading back, Andy came by and informed us that he was not sure if the water in the streams we had passed would be safe to drink or not. Then again, at this point, it's probably better to hydrate than to die. Comforting, eh?

Soon after that encounter with Andy, Joe came back with Damien and he called us out for not keeping pace. Behind him, the rest of the teams of racers came up and soon we were back in the race with everyone else.

It turned out that while we were busy dragging that damn tire through 18 miles of Hell, there was a swim challenge that we had missed, at this point it no longer mattered. Joe instructed us to simply continue. Since they caught us on our way back to the tire, they had us carry-on with that objective and we all headed back to the spot where we dropped the tire off.

Once we got back to the tire, we had more burpees – 100 to

be exact. As soon as all of Team Ten made it back to the tire, our team was punished for not making it as a team to the swim. Our punishment? The race directors sent us back to carrying that damn tire. We had hoped that our reuniting with the rest of the Death Racers would shed a spark in others to help our cause. Our hopes of the other teams helping us were all for not. It was upsetting, but there was nothing we could do but carry-on.

All of us tried to organize a system to move the tire efficiently, but almost instantaneously I became annoyed. Every method we had attempted to implement up until now was less effective than we had hoped, since we spent most of our time with the tire on single track trails. The most infuriating part of returning to the tire was dealing with the dichotomy of the group's work ethic. Half of the group would step up more often to take turns on the tire while others made what seemed to be a purposeful effort to slip to the back of the pack right before it was their turn on the tire. This happened more times than it should have.

Eventually, people called each other out and the problem appeared to be solved, but it was only temporary. Team Ten was still mighty, but we had our troubles. We tried to keep up with the other racers, but all they had to carry were their packs. Meanwhile, we had our large rucks and this cursed tire to drag. Trying to keep up was a lost cause, but as we made our way back to the farm, we would occasionally approach other racers who stopped to refill their water from some of the runoff streams on the mountainside. To purify the water most of us utilized iodine tabs, which meant a minimum of 30 minutes before drinking the water.

Every so often a few racers would pass us by as we dragged the tire and we would realize that we were still in this. By the time we made it out of the woods and all the nasty spots, we had finally deployed a superior system for dragging the tire. It took a while for us to develop this solution, but that's what it is all about, trial and error and figuring things out. Just because we were being challenged and we were dealt an unfair card did not mean we could give up, we had to keep our heads up and focus on completing the challenges we were given, regardless of what everyone else had to do in the race.

The system that we eventually developed utilized a series of ropes that were strategically attached to the tire with other lines connected to the main ones to create branches. All of these cords and ropes allowed us to have more than six people pulling at any given time. With the tire dragging behind us, we eventually emerged from the trail and found ourselves on a paved road with a house at the trailhead.

There, we were treated by the owner of the house to free water from his hose. This was an incredibly exciting moment for us. Though after a short reprieve, we were back at it with that tire. Soon we found ourselves faced with another fork in the road and, undecided on which way would lead us back to Amee Farm, we began to argue amongst ourselves about our options and why one way was better than the other. The homeowner tried to offer us some seemingly helpful information, but we had to consider the circumstances of this year's theme, which left us uncertain we could trust the source. We did not know who he was; we did not know if he was in on the race or if he was merely a local that wanted to be helpful. We just didn't know.

The **Year of Betrayal** theme made it difficult for us to discern between who and what to trust. With every passing minute of the race, our ability to trust anyone, even ourselves, diminished. Furthermore, we still had no idea which way to go.

CHAPTER 6

HUMAN ERROR OR BETRAYAL?

"Doing just a little bit during the time we have available puts you that much further ahead than if you took no action at all." ~ Pulsifer

Halted by another fork in the road, everyone on the team disputed the information we had received from a few different sources. Throughout our treks we would encounter other racers, volunteers and other people involved in the race, and oftentimes you found yourself questioning who had the factual knowledge to get you where you needed to be. A few members insisted we go one way, while others favored the other path, and the remainder were perplexed as to how we wound up in this pickle.

Although it took over 30 minutes to make a decision, everyone was provided an opportunity to voice their opinion which eventually led to an agreement on which direction we should head. When you are traveling in groups this large, it becomes more and more difficult to get group consensus, on top of that you are starting to deal with sleep deprivation, these two things put a massive strain on the human's ability to not only make a decision but also be confident in that decision. Decisions that should happen in an instant can and will drag on. After the debate was over, we turned around and made our way back to the last intersection we had passed, maybe an eighth of a mile back. We truly hoped that route would be the fastest way back to Amee Farm.

Once again, it was us against the tire, but at least now we had a solidified system for effectively and efficiently moving all 500 pounds of tire. With a combination of ropes and webbing we effectively created a series of handles affixed to this massive tire and with some athletes carrying multiple rucks, others focused on pulling while the rest pushed from behind, we navigated these roads with ease. And that was just it, now that we were on wide open, actual roads, we had all the room we needed to utilize all of our strength to travel faster, safer. No more using only a tenth of our strength at a time. Even when we had to move aside for cars, this was a far better situation than what we had been subjected to for countless hours the night before. The ultimate relief, however, came from the shift in overall group morale, the arguments and tensions finally subsided. Hours ago we were a shit show, but now? Now, we were doing quite marvelous, really!

Thankfully, some of our teammates' crew members showed up and helped us to replenish a few of the countless calories and fluids we lost over the course of the past 24 hours. The best food item from the everyone-grab-what-you-can free-for-all was the clementines. They were so damn delicious. With our bodies refueled and a decision on which direction to go, we collectively decided that no matter what, we would finish this race, even if we had to drag that tire for another 48 hours to do so. That is how determined and dedicated we grew to be during our time together.

We looked like a ragged band of misfits, charging down the road with a massive tractor tire in tow, we were down to roughly fourteen members, on our team. As far was we were concerned we were still in this race. Some of our teammates were breaking down, their bodies just couldn't handle it. You could see it in their eyes, that look of defeat. While they were still moving along and going through the motion, you could see their effort was diminishing. Slowly but surely they were giving up, their race was seemingly coming to an end. This is no fault of their own, some of them simply weren't as physically prepared as they thought they were, others had merely aggravated old injuries and then there were the unlucky few who developed new injuries since the beginning of the event. While they had come far, the race was taking its toll. It was quickly devouring the underprepared and the over-ambitious.

As we continued to move as a unified group with that massive tire, we rounded a few corners, ascended and descended a few hills, and pushed forward with determination. Soon, we came upon the peak of a particular hill as we dragged the tire down the middle of the road and when we reached the crest, we could see a group of racers led by Joe. To this day, I wish I could have captured a picture of that moment, or better yet a video. Where's that iPhone when you need it? This moment was so vivid and memorable that I can still see it with full clarity in my mind. After all these years, it still stands out to this day.

Joe had this look of astonishment on his face. It was a look of disbelief like he couldn't believe we all had smiles on our faces after dragging this blasted tire around. The look said, "Holy shit these mofo's won't quit. What do I do to them?" and it was glorious. It was staggering to see that look of fear that we would not be broken glimmer in Joe's eyes. He quickly fixed his composure, so fast I am not sure anyone else witnessed that same moment of shock that I did.

Without skipping a beat, Joe fired off a bunch of threats that our team was so far behind we could never finish. He told us we could not finish. He told us we could not go on. He told us we were done. A few of us rebuked his sentiments posthaste.

We told Joe, "No, we are not finished. We are not done with this race. We will go on, regardless. We will drag this damn tire the entire race if we have to. WE. ARE. FINISHING!"

Joe collected himself and told our crew members that we could not continue dragging this tire around any longer if we insisted on staying in the race. He asked some people that were with him if they could see to it that the tire would make it back to Amee Farm.

From here on out we were free of the tire.

After more than 20 hours with the tire and more than 24 hours of racing as a team, in an instant, we were no longer on the same team. It was finally time for this event to become an individual race. To be clear, the Death Race still isn't technically a race by your typical standards. With all the unknown variables, the lack of a physical start or finish line, and all the moments in which participants are required to work together; it is difficult to declare the Death Race an actual race. It is much more of a challenge with elements of a traditional race sprinkled throughout the event.

For our next task, we were to head over to Joe's residence. We started running with the rest of the racers that followed behind Joe and we all made our way back toward his property. I made sure to stay near the front of the pack; I refused to fall behind any more than we already had. For my comfort, I tried to stick with people I knew, so once I had spotted a few familiar faces I said hello and we continued on our way back past the fork of indecision from earlier.

This time, since we were following behind Joe, there was no hesitation on which way to go. This time we took the alternate path. When we arrived at Joe's property, we had to perform the plank position on a hill. We positioned ourselves on the decline of the slope with our heads faced toward the bottom were Joe stood. There we waited for everyone else to arrive and join us, as we held, and held, and held.

In this moment, it did not pay to be in the lead, being in the lead meant you were now forced to hold a plank for a longer period of time than those who are a bit slower and arrived moments later – to me, this was a lesson learned! Three minutes later, everyone had finally made it and we continued to hold that plank. Everyone would occasionally tap a knee at this point, but they would quickly resume holding until Joe decided it was time to move on out. Holding that plank was challenging, but it was just a small part of this enormous undertaking and did little to discourage my spirits.

On our way to the next challenge, I remember we made our

way up a path next to Joe's where another fork split the trail. As you would expect, some participants chose one pathway while the rest wanted the other. For whatever reason, I second-guessed my decision within a few 100 feet and doubled back to take the alternate route. I would soon find out that it did not matter which route was taken; both trails led to the same location.

Upon our arrival, we were presented with an interesting challenge. Racers were partnered up into a few small teams that varied in size anywhere from two people to a group of five. This task led to what many would argue was "cheating" but I write this in quotes because it is highly-debatable what happened. Four of us were placed in a group together and to be honest, I was going through some crazy fatigue and began a downward spiral that would lead my mind to the dangerous thought of

Q.

U.

I.

T.

T.

I.

N.

G.

Yes, quitting.

When it comes to quitting, the knowledge that I had collected over the years from experience and watching others, is that when you start letting negative thoughts into your head, they can quickly compound themselves. They will proliferate until you either give in to the notion or break the darkness and persevere.

For example, back when I was a gymnast one of the primary things we were taught was to visualize our routines in their entirety all the way down to the execution of your salute at the beginning and end of the routine. The idea is that if you visualize yourself executing each move with perfect form, you are that much more likely to do so when you go up on the apparatus to perform. When I imagined myself falling, or saw myself making a mistake in my head, more often than not, I fell off or made some sort of mistake. I knew the power of a positive mindset and simply thinking positively is what I needed to do to stop myself from thinking about doing something as stupid as quitting. Visualize, then, execute. That's what I needed to do. See myself finishing, see myself earning my skull.

Once we were in our groups, we were assigned buckets to fill with gravel. Those buckets would then need to be brought up the mountain trail to pour out on various bike trails. Our team was designated with the number 32 and it was required that we find a stake in the ground with that number written on it.

My shoulder felt wrecked. The treacherous tractor tire did a number on me. The thought of carrying a bucket seemed impossible. Pain radiated from the tear in my labrum, there wasn't a moment during the event that it did not hurt. Most of the time, I did everything in my power to mentally compartmentalize that pain and put it somewhere else. The reality was, hiking around with a 40-50 lb ruck, carrying heavy objects, pushing and pulling that tire through Bloodroot and beyond, I started to wonder how much longer my torn shoulder would hold up.

I stood there for a minute and wondered if I could go on without doing irreparable damage. They were checking the fill height of everyone's buckets. I couldn't bring back a half-empty bucket. I looked to my teammates and explained to them what was going on with the tear in my shoulder. I told them how I did not want to skimp out on the labor, but it was clear that we would have to make at least two trips up the mountain and there were four of us. Each of us could only carry one full bucket at a time.

I suggested, to maximize our effectiveness, that while they were moving the buckets, I could run faster and search all the different trails for these numbered trail marking sticks. Without a complaint, they agreed, and I cannot thank those guys enough for helping me out by going along with this strategy. I truly appreciate what that did for the group and myself; it was us against the race, if we were all in "the suck" of it together, we might as well help each other through.

According to Urban Dictionary, "The Suck" can be defined as the Unofficial slang term used by the Marine Corps. It defines any situation in and around a wartime conflict where conditions are undesirable. Also known as "The Shit."

While we obviously were not in a wartime conflict, the conditions we endured were far less than desirable.

I took off but hit another fatigued moment as I tried to make my way up the mountain. I sat down on a rock and started scouring through my bag for something to eat. In the depths of my ruck, I found a bag that was about a quarter of the way full of pretzels. I started eating them quickly. Just then, Todd was making his way up, and I offered some to him. He was in a hurry to finish this challenge, so Todd made sure I was doing alright and quickly carried on. After a couple of minutes, I slurped down my last GU packet and went back to searching for the number 32 stick. I found a bunch of numbers. Team 5, Team 42, 38, etc. Everywhere I looked I found trail marking sticks with every number except the one I needed. Some of them positioned close to where the bike trails started and others near the top of the mountain; some were as far up as the cabin where we weighed in at the start of the event.

After searching for a considerable amount of time, I ran back to the bottom to report my status to the rest of my team. The team was readying themselves to bring the next round of buckets up. I told them I would continue to look. I saw Todd again and asked him what team number he was as he hadn't found his team's stick. I was hoping for his sake maybe one of the ones I saw corresponded with his team number. Things got quite confusing when he responded, "I'm team 32."

I immediately responded, "Get out of here, we're team 32. Are you sure?" I ran back down to check with the race volunteers who were tracking this objective. I explained to the volunteer the issue and he said it was impossible.

Was this a betrayal? Were all the trail marking sticks out there merely random numbers and no one could find their numbered stick? No, I did come across a few groups that found their stick. Did some racers take other teams' sticks and change them to their number? Unfortunately, yes. I saw this happen a few times. So what happened to ours? Did it exist?

Well, I went back and told my teammates and Todd about the current situation. I headed off to look for our stick, while I did that, I believe Todd decided just to make one of his own by betraying someone else's. When I got back down, I was informed by someone's crew member, Andy Greenwood, that our situation was explained to the volunteers by both teams. They admitted they must have made a mistake and told us we were free to move on to the next challenge.

It was all very confusing, I no longer knew what was actually a part of the race, what was a deception, and what was simply a big mistake. For all I knew, this could have all been part of their elaborate plan, or they were just careless and made some mistakes. Admittedly, I was frustrated by the thought that they might make these types of mistakes, but I tried not to think about it too much. There was no time for being frustrated, what mattered was moving forward to whatever was next.

Andy G. was kind enough to hang back to make sure I knew I could move on to the next task. He asked me if there was anything he could do to help me since I had still not met up with Jennifer, my only crew member. I was out of my pain medicine, so until I made it back to Mark's car I would be in a lot of pain. Andy G. said he would do his best to find Adam, or Mark and ultimately my medicine.

Although my shoulder was going to suffer for a while, I was happy to hear that I could stop looking for the stick. The sun was making its way down into the mountains and soon it would be dark. I would not want to search for a stake at night with only the light of my headlamp to guide me. I made my way back down the hill to where all these massive logs were lined up along the sides of the road. I was instructed to find a log and join the rest of the racers. We were to split our log in half and then both halves into sixths.

Finally, relief from carrying my pack, relief from running up and down hills. The idea of chopping wood for a while made me happy. Time to rip off my compression shirt and get out my beloved Fiskars x27 splitting ax, and of course, recite a song from my childhood in my head as I chopped away.

What rolls down stairs

alone or in pairs,

and over your neighbor's dog?

What's great for a snack,

And fits on your back?

It's a log, log, log

It's log; it's log,

It's big; it's heavy, it's wood.

It's log; it's log, it's better than bad, it's good.

Everyone wants a log

You're gonna love it, log

Come on and get your log

Everyone needs a log

log log log

Good old Ren & Stimpy, it's a classic, one that I couldn't resist remembering at a time like this. It was helpful to my mindset. It made me, happy. I was in a good place, chopping wood.

CHAPTER 7

MAKE IT HURT SO GOOD

"Nothing can stop the man with the right mental attitude from achieving his goal; nothing on earth can help the man with the wrong mental attitude." ~ Thomas Jefferson

Finally, I had the chance to get a reprieve from carrying my pack. I was overdue to give my shoulder rest from all of the added weight. Unfortunately, the next task involved swinging an ax, and being that I am left-handed and the tear was in my left shoulder, splitting a log into halves and then sixths was not the kind of rest my shoulder needed.

I walked along the right side of the road and all along the roadside there appeared to be a fresh delivery of cut trees and logs, all of which needed a thorough chopping. Earlier, when we came through this area for check-in, the logs were not here, at least not from what I could recall. I immediately searched for a log that was substantial but manageable.

As I scoured the area for the "right" log to chop, I came to a few quick realizations. First, the easy pickin's were becoming scarce at an alarming rate. Second, some of these logs were GINORMOUS! The last realization I had was the extent to which I had aggravated my injured shoulder. It had become a serious issue and I needed to be even more conscientious of it from here on out.

I would have to chop this log using both right and left handed swings to get through the challenge; one should do that anyway when chopping to keep the workload balanced. I found a log with a diameter slightly larger, by about half a foot, than I would have liked, but there was no time to be picky. I grasped the log tightly and pulled it onto the road. Finding some open space, I made an area all for myself to start chopping.

Even though I had cleared an area, I was very nervous about how close people would walk within my swinging radius. It seemed like no one was mindful of the wildly swinging axes, this included racers, volunteers, and support crew members. It was quite the scene; there was this sea of people, all hacking away at their logs on this fire road in the middle of the woods. Chips and splinters of wood whizzed by your face and everywhere you looked you feared for the escalating likelihood that something could go very wrong, very quickly.

Navigating this dangerous maze had me frightened, but I kept myself collected. A few racers broke their ax heads off. Others struggled to get their ax to split through all the way; often you would see athletes take out their hand saws to finish getting through their log. The open spot I thought I had cleared for myself continued to be a nuisance for me. After changing the angle from which I swung my ax, I became more relaxed, though the fear of hitting someone was still very real.

Smack, crack.

Smack, smack, crack.

Smack, crack, clunk, clunk.

All you heard all around you were the sounds of axes ripping through the logs and their pieces hitting the ground. Wood splinters flew off in every direction. After every 10-20 strikes or so, I would take a pause, switch dominant arms and go back to swinging. I positioned my log with a rock wedged in front of it to minimize its rolling and movement.

Trying to get this log in half was quite the task, there was a pretty nasty knot toward the center. And while I didn't have exactly a one-swing split, it only took a few strikes before my first half divided. Soon enough I had my first six splits, and I was ready to move onto the other half.

Once I had a dozen pieces of firewood, it was time to strategize. The next part of this challenge was to return to Amee Farm. As I recall, a few people were sent back to the Farm and were told to leave their wood. They had to serve a penalty for the "cheating" that happened during the hunt for the numbered sticks.

Their punishment? Tread water in the pond for varied amounts of time. Our situation was different because of the mistakes the volunteers made, so we were given the go-ahead and did not have to join them.

I stayed behind with a few other fellow racers to figure out how I would get all these logs back in a way that would not add to all the pain that my shoulder was experiencing. If there was ever a time I could have used my pain medicine, it was right then. If I had more pills readily available at this point, the following events may have unraveled quite differently.

For some time I played around with different configurations. I strapped all my logs to my Gunslinger rucksack. That was a fail. When I tried to stand, with all the weight of my ruck and the log, I could barely get my pack off the ground. So then, I split the load in half, I tried putting six logs in my bucket and strapping the other six to my pack. Another fail as I still couldn't bear that much weight on my shoulder.

What was I to do?

The sun was gone. The dark of night covered the floor of the forest. With the darkness upon us, I found myself teaming up with a fellow racer. The two of us spent some time grabbing a few long, skinny trees from the wooded areas next to the fire road. Once our materials were sourced, we proceeded to build a sled of sorts. We utilized a lot of rope to bundle the logs, and even more 550 paracord to create a platform and tension system that would hopefully hold everything together.

To our dismay, all that effort was a waste of our energy, strength, and time. The sled did not work at all and it fell apart within seconds. Our brains were not functioning at their full potential. We should have known that wouldn't have worked, but we were willing to try anything to ease the workload.

It wasn't going to be simple, it was going to be evil, so heinous that it would eat at me and put me into a downward spiral that would lead to my first real desire to just quit the damn race. The harsh reality I now faced was the fact I didn't have the power I needed to accomplish this task as easily as I would without a torn shoulder.

Since the sled did not work, I decided there was no way around it; I was going to have to take two trips to get all the wood down to the farm. As I recall, it would be an 8-mile round trip, which I would have to do twice. That is a lot of ground to cover just to finish what should be accomplishable in one go. I reluctantly dropped half of my logs.

I scooped the other half up and made my way out with Patrick W. and another racer. We began our descent and my bundle did not want to cooperate with me. It would not stay together regardless of what efforts I made to force it to remain a unit. Some pieces would slide out, which forced me to make frequent adjustments.

Thankfully, Patrick lent me some compression straps, which made things a lot more bearable. My shoulder continued to aggravate me. In an ideal world, I would have been better off if I could take my mind elsewhere and not think about it, but as much as I tried to distract my mind from the pain, nothing could hold my attention long enough to stop my mind from converging on the agony I felt.

As we descended the mountain with our logs, we came across another group of racers including Morgan. Morgan is a fellow Storm Chaser that I knew from a brief meeting nearly six months prior when I traveled to the World Championship Spartan Race in Glen Rose, Texas for my 26th birthday. I was excited to see a familiar face. We bonded right away over a discussion about how unforgiving this race was and how deep in "the suck" it put us. The reality is, we were both aggravated by how things were going.

The notion of quitting lingered and began to seep into my soul, trying to control my mind as my thoughts focused on the quantity of suck that I had already endured. Then, I realized how much more there was still to come. It quickly spiraled. It became one negative thought after the other.

This is pointless. I am hurt.

How severe would my pain be had I not had that cortisone shot the Monday before the race?

Why am I here? Should I even bother finishing this race? Should WE even bother?

I was losing focus on the goals I had set before starting the race. I no longer cared if I finished or not. I thought about how I was actually very proud of how far I had come. Finishing seemed so far away and some of the insanity of this twisted race was getting the best of us. Under the darkness of the night, the silence of the forest, and the pain....the...

Oh

My

GOD!

The PAIN!

The pain had become so unbearable that I just could not do this anymore.

"Fuck this and fuck that," is all I thought and said.

I did not want to do this race anymore.

I QUIT!

These thoughts and emotions poured out. I'd had it – and I wasn't the only one. Soon enough, Morgan and I had both made the same decision. We decided, *you know what sounds a lot better than this madness...a beer!*

That's right, Morgan and I had agreed. This was it. We were going to quit and become TEAM BEER! While everyone else would continue to suffer, we would go and grab a beer and have fun during our remaining time in Vermont. We chucked our wood into the forest and I returned Patrick's compression straps.

When I told him, he was a bit shocked. Patrick didn't blame us. He felt this year's race was way different from last year when he finished. Patrick expressed to us that he was not having as good of an experience as he remembered having a year prior and even he had considered throwing in the towel. I am happy to say, he never did. Patrick was an inspiring person out there. I am so glad we worked together here and on Team Tire.

Even though Morgan and I had decided we were done, we still had over three miles to get back to the farm. Those three miles were some of the most absurdly dark and technical we would face. Due to the lack of sleep, we were beginning to experience the consequences of sleep deprivation. Once we had an understanding of the path to take back, Morgan and I decided we were going to break off from Patrick and the others, so we could get back faster. The path zigged and zagged. There were a few long switchbacks we traveled down when Morgan had the most peculiar hallucination. "Is that the Michelin Man?" she questioned.

Perplexed, I looked at Morgan and back out into the woods. I did not see the Michelin Man, but I did see what she was talking about. It was another racer not too far off in the distance. The lack of sleep was really doing a number on what we perceived ahead as we hiked along that path.

With the darkness and how far off the trail we went since we split off from Patrick we found ourselves a little lost looking for the steel I-beam bridge that crossed Tweed River and lead back to the trail to Amee Farm. Since we couldn't seem to find the steel beam to get back across we opted to just suck it up and cross the shallow river together. Once we made it across to the other side, we had to go through a field of tall, wet grass. At the time, I was only wearing a pair of shorts, a compression shirt, and a set of calf compression sleeves. My legs were already wet and cold from walking across the creek. The damp grass made it feel colder than it really was and added to the suck of it all.

All I wanted was to get out of that field. In the distance we could see a faint light shining and we had hoped that it was Amee Farm. It wasn't. When we made it back to Route 100, the main road to town, we looked left, and we looked right, and we had no clue where we were. With a lingering feeling of helplessness, we plopped ourselves down in front of a house that sold Maple Syrup, as advertised by the sign outside the building. I took out my phone and tried to see if I could get any signal but sadly, there was none.

My body temperature started to drop. I began to shiver. The two of us huddled close and thankfully, Morgan pulled out a foil blanket. Together, we wrapped ourselves in the foil blanket as Morgan searched her bag for her fire starter. Within a few short minutes, we had a mini fire burning on the side of the road as we snacked on some trail mix, pretzels, and I even had a piece of chocolate, which is a rare treat for me. That little bit of chocolate brought some life back into me.

As we sat there bundled up next to our puny little fire, a few cars drove past. Every time we saw a car, we would start waving a twig that was lit on fire, and I would move my bright iPhone screen in hopes that someone would stop. Not once did it cross our minds that the drivers all probably think these two people on the side of the road are absolutely nuts. Two people, wrapped up in a foil blanket waving a cell phone and a twig that's on fire at passersby. It was clear that our brains were fried and we were not making the best decisions.

After many ill attempts, more than I expected would be possible at 4 AM, to get a lift from a passing car we decided it was time to pack our food and supplies back up. Now that we had time to warm up and recover some calories, we had to start moving. I was confident that the road we were one was the main Route 100 that runs through the town of Pittsfield, and given that, I assumed we only had to go about a mile to get back to Amee Farm.

Sure enough, as the sun rose behind the mountains and

it dimly lit the sky, I could see just down the road — there it was! Amee Farm. As we got even closer, I could see someone running across the street. I knew within a tenth of a second who it was, "Norm?!" I shouted, hoping I wasn't wrong. He saw us and once he realized who it was asked why the hell we were coming from that direction. We explained how we were lost and wanted to throw in the towel. I could tell he was disappointed to hear that, but he also seemed very eager to bring us to Andy to report this news. Was he one of the moles?

Norm brought us over to Andy. We said to him, "Andy, I think we're done. I think we are done with this."

The red LED lights on the timer displayed how long the race had been going. I think it read around 38 hours and some minutes.

"We've already been in this race for 38 hours," I had thought to myself. That's pretty damn incredible given that before this the longest challenge I completed lasted a mere thirteen hours or so.

Andy's response left me shocked. From everything I knew about the race, and especially about quitting the race. What Andy said to us next was not what you would expect to hear from the Race Director. Typically, they encouraged quitting at this race. Andy looked at both of us, and with a deep concern for how far we had already made it, he asked us, "Are you sure?"

CHAPTER 8

THE COMEBACK KIDS

"If you don't risk anything, you risk even more." ~ Erica Jong

Andy asked me whether I was sure I wanted to quit or not. Well no, I was not sure that I wanted to quit. The reality was that I wanted more than anything to finish. After all, that's why I came out to Vermont to compete in this race in the first place. I wanted to see what I was made of. Until these moments of self-doubt, finishing the Death Race was the only option I had ever considered.

Days before the race I took my lunch break at work to sit down and pull a Bart Simpson with the whiteboard and wrote: "I will finish the Death Race" until I covered the entire dry erase board. When Andy offered me the moment to decide if I really wanted to quit I knew I had to re-evaluate the situation at hand. Morgan suggested she was feeling the need to reconsider her position whether to continue participating or not.

That one question made us rethink every thought we had about quitting throughout the night. Now with a new day upon us, and Andy's "Are you sure you want to quit?" question lingering, all it took was a quick look at each other and then back at Andy.

We responded together, "Give us a few to think this through."

I looked over at a nearby fire pit. It was hard to tell but I saw what appeared to be my friend, Jennifer, she was lying there on a makeshift cot made from a couple of chairs. At long last, I finally had the opportunity to see my one crew member. When I saw Jennifer, I wanted to tell her immediately about how I had considered quitting. But I also really didn't want to tell her that I even harbored the thought.

She appeared to be only half awake when I approached, but when I got up close to her, I could see that she was out cold. She came to and I quickly explained to her the situation with my shoulder. I told her how Andy was questioning our desire to quit. She told me that no matter what choice I made, that I had to be proud of how far I had come. She was, and so was I. But still, I was only half satisfied. After all, I don't like quitting.

Jennifer invited me to join her for a bit in the makeshift cot to warm up. Thankfully, though she looked cold, she was quite warm. She placed my legs under her sleeping bag and provided me with a warmth I very much needed. Just that combination of body heat and the sleeping bag brought all the warmth back to my body. It was nice. I was feeling better already.

Before sitting down, I had taken a moment to remove my shoes and socks, placing them by the fire to let them dry. With my need for warmth met, I could focus on another unsettling and rather inevitable reality – I was starving!

I'm not sure what my calorie deficit was at this point in the race, but in a 100 mile running race I would burn somewhere between 12,500 and 15,000 calories, based on the amount of calories I typically burn per mile. If I calculate everything I had eaten up to that point, I was easily in the 10,000 calorie deficit range.

The lack of calories was not helping to make the decision of whether or not I wanted to carry-on any simpler. To feed my depleted body, Jennifer whipped out several MRE (Meal, Ready to Eat) packs and started feeding me. I enjoyed an oatmeal cookie that I lathered with peanut butter and after that chowed down on some roasted almonds. Let me tell you, those simple pleasures were absolutely delightful!

Jennifer explained to me how she spent the evening waiting there keeping her eye out for me from the time she arrived. It turned out that she was informed racers would eventually be making their way back to the farm. Instead of searching for me on the mountain and missing me, she decided to wait at the farm; the plan was to link up with me when I returned.

Well, it turned out that between the time she received that information and I actually arrived was quite a long while. Jennifer spent her entire night lying on that makeshift cot calling out for me. She would call out my name over and over throughout the night. Because of the darkness out in Vermont, it was difficult to identify faces so she would shout out *"Tony?!"* to over 30 people who came through before me.

Jennifer called out to every one of them in hopes of finding me. Someone actually responded one of the times, but it was the wrong Tony. Having a friend that is willing to spend that kind of time helping you achieve your dreams is instrumental in making these endeavors that much more manageable. People like Jennifer are angels on earth, I cannot thank her enough for sacrificing the hours of sleep and time she did just to make sure she didn't miss me coming through. These are the kind of people you want in your life. People who lift you up and support your dreams.

As life returned to me, I got up and told Jennifer I would be back in a bit. I went over to the racer's tent to see Morgan. She was organizing some things and had decided she wanted to continue on. She started hounding me to come with and finish what we started. Initially, I was still uncertain. My shoulder was radiating with pain!

I asked Morgan to give me a few more minutes to make my decision and for a moment, I thought I had an idea. I scrambled from the tent and went to Andy. I couldn't carry the wood, but maybe I could negotiate some sort of alternative obstacle. Andy wasn't buying it, though. I had to bring the logs back to the farm. He liked where my head was at, but if I didn't bring the logs down, I was done.

So I paused and I thought some more.

I thought about how Andy, who has completed some of the most extreme events out there in his own life, must have dealt with injuries before. I asked him to be straight-up with me about my shoulder tear and what he thought I should do. He told me ultimately I have to decide. If I thought this could cause permanent damage, lifelong damage, if I thought that were possible, I should really take that into consideration when making my decision. I didn't have much time left to think. This was a race, and if I wanted a shot at finishing, I had to get moving!

With this new advice, my mind was made up, I was not ready to quit. Of course, I was also not fully prepared to go back to those logs. Another twelve to sixteen miles would await me. Just to finish a challenge I was only three miles away from completing half of before I decided I wanted to quit. The thought of how I shouldn't have done that lurked in the corner of my thoughts, poking me over and over to remind me not to give up so easily ever again.

While I contemplated my decision, off in the distance, I saw Todd. He was making some adjustments before heading back out to his next challenge. I gave him a quick rundown and asked his advice. He looked at me and then divulged to me the key element that would make this race beatable.

We had gone over whether or not I could feasibly go back up the mountain and bring at the very least a couple logs at a time. Of course, I could handle that – other than a couple blisters starting to form on the ball of my foot I felt pretty golden. It was just the thought of excessive weight in addition to the weight of the pack that got to me. Todd suggested that no one said you have to take the logs down all at once. If you must, then simply take one at a time. Good logic right?

It would be more distance but, I would still be in the race. That wasn't the key piece of advice, though. That came next when Todd said to me, "Only you can pull yourself from this race."

Only I could pull myself from the race?

He was right, there were no real disqualifications. That was part of the mental game. If we truly wanted to continue on and continue racing, who was going to stop us?

No one.

Not Joe.

Not Andy.

Not any volunteer.

The only person who could disqualify you from the race was yourself. You are your own worst enemy.

With this new found knowledge, I thanked Todd a thousand times over and gave my favorite red-headed giant a hug, wishing him the best of luck with the rest of his race.

When I first heard of the Death Race, I planned to compete for the first time in 2013, but one of the main reasons I was here racing in 2012 instead of waiting until 2013 was because of this guy. Todd has a way of motivating and inspiring that is unparalleled. Hell, the man often claimed that training for the Death Race is a crutch, and while I disagreed, in a lot of ways, he was right.

I shuffled my way through the wet grass back over to Morgan in the racers' tent. I sat down with her and asked if she was going to continue on. I told her my shoulder was in agony and it made things extremely difficult, but if I had to go one log at a time then maybe I could continue on. For some time she had been harping on about how we couldn't quit.

"Are you going to keep harassing me until I decide to keep going?" I questioned her.

Morgan's head nodded up and down and she vocally confirmed that she would not let me quit.

Well, alright then, "Let's do this damn thing!" I exclaimed.

By the time we had our gear back together and acknowledged our desire to continue the red led lights of the LED race clock displayed just over 40 hours elapsed. Jennifer wished me good luck and told me she would keep in contact with my dad about my progress. During the prep time just before we set back out on the trails, I ran over to Mark's car in hopes of finding his keys in his bumper. I searched and searched but couldn't find anything. Then I heard a noise. I started to walk toward the rear passenger door when a head shot up and I jumped back.

It was Mark. I was shocked. He quickly handed me my container of pain medicine as he opened the door. Apparently, my message traveled well through the Death Race community. Unfortunately for Mark, he almost destroyed his Achilles and had to bow out. His doctor would later confirm that it was a very wise decision on his part to pull out of the race when he did.

Mark unfortunately "DNF'd" this Death Race (DNF is short for "did not finish"). He bowed-out a few hours prior but assured me he would hang out until I was finished. For that I was immensely grateful, the last thing I would want to do after not finishing a race is hang around.

With my belly full, my body warmed, the bright rays of the morning sun shining bright, my headspace realigned, and all the pills I might need, Morgan and I eagerly grabbed our gear and headed back on the trail. The two of us felt refreshed and silly for wanting to quit. We hustled our way from the farm towards the mountain once again. We had some options for which direction we could take to get back to where we chopped the wood. There was the standard trail route, which would probably consume more time over a longer distance.

Alternatively, we could head up the ravine. It was a bit more challenging and involved the likeliness of getting our feet wet again. However, it would decrease the amount of distance we would have to travel and hopefully, the amount of time as well. This is where I discovered that the shoe I chose as my second pair would not be to my benefit.

I had chosen to bring along my New Balance MT10's as

my second pair of shoes. The problem with the MT10's was that they were near the end of their lifespan. They had been through quite a few races, many runs, and a few other miscellaneous adventures. Though the bottoms were low on traction, I don't think it was the fault of them being old. The ravine was slippery, and wet rocks tended to be even more so. This is what made this route a bit more dangerous. I found myself landing on my ass more than a few times, and every time I slipped, Morgan and I laughed it up. The daylight made things less miserable and the suck became more enjoyable, that or perhaps we were just loopy from the lack of sleep.

It didn't matter that my shoes were slippery, tractionless, death traps. The sun was shining through the trees as the water trickled down the ravine, everything around me seemed oh so serene. It was pure bliss. This was the life. This was some damn good living!

It is still a wonder to me how refreshing and revitalizing the sun can be. As we bathed ourselves in Vitamin D, it was as if the sun reinvigorated our very souls and gave us that extra push to be happy about racing again. There was nothing that could wipe the big smiles off our faces. We were back in the Death Race, and we had decided to make a pact. From here on out we would finish this race. Together, we would finish the Death Race. No matter what. Together, we would be unbreakable.

CHAPTER 9

AND WE'LL KEEP ON FIGHTING TIL THE END

The most common way people give up their power is by thinking they don't have any." ~ Alice Walker

Being out on the mountain, living, surviving, embracing the challenges both physically and mentally pushed all of us to become better versions of ourselves. This is what life should be about for those seeking to get more out of themselves.

Adventure.

Challenges.

Having the courage to take on the unexpected.

From chaos, came clarity.

From the jaws of defeat, I found the strength to go on – I found a strange sense of happiness.

My friend Morgan and I discovered the inner strength to push on. Camaraderie creates a powerful connection. It can make the impossible seem like just another training day. As a young, single 20-something year old, the presence of a strong, powerful woman not only supplied me with plenty of male machismo, but it also gave me the will and strength to embrace the task of continuing on with this race.

I remember Morgan telling me about an incident early-on when she was dehydrated and found herself vomiting. I was thankful, for both our sake, that she recovered because the way I see it, without her, continuing may not have happened. In many ways her presence gave me the courage to go on.

Halfway up a ravine, the two of us found a couple of bundles of what appeared to be pre-split logs. Upon further investigation, we discovered not only where they already split logs, but there were 12 of them. This could be our first six out of twelve, we both thought. Morgan suggested we move forward and continue to the top of the ravine to see if anyone was making their way back.

We met a trio of racers, but they were already on to another challenge.

This was...perfect.

We could head back down and save ourselves time traveling back to our previously split leftovers. And if we couldn't find them, it would have been worse to need to chop more wood. From there, we immediately pulled a 180° back down the ravine. Once we had made it back to the spot where we found the new logs, I managed to squeeze six of them into my bucket. Morgan stuffed the other six in her pack.

I had removed my rucksack and only brought my bucket up. It seemed wise to stash my ruck at the bottom in a nook out of a fear of having my gear hijacked. Given the theme of betrayal, I had no concept of exactly how risky this might be. Nevertheless, I was willing to take the gamble to give my shoulder the relief I would need before what I assumed might be the very real possibility of splitting more wood.

It was a safe bet as the pack went untouched.

During the descent, we went slightly off-course to avoid the ravine. Truth be told, I had grown sick and tired of falling on my ass and looking like a fool during the ascent. I took off ahead so I could retrieve my pack. Finding the right place to cut-back into the ravine to the nook's location required a few pauses so I could regain my bearings, but it wasn't long before I found it. Once I recovered the pack, I made my way back to meet Morgan on the elevated path that followed the nearby ravine we previously struggled to traverse.

Without the burden of carrying my pack for the first section of the descent made it easier and I was far enough ahead that I had a moment to sit down.

Bad idea, soon enough I was fading away.

Snap! Crack!

Huh?

What?

My heart began to beat rapidly. It wasn't so much fear as it was panic that woke me. I worried about another racer, or worse, a volunteer or race director finding me asleep. When I think back, it seems kind of silly, considering that at that moment in the race we were closing in on 42-hours of racing not including the time awake before the race started.

The thought was mind-numbing. I had already been awake for two days.

"Damn," I thought. "That's a lot of hours of consecutive activity."

I grabbed my pack, stood up, then Morgan and I continued. We reached a series of switchbacks that led us down the mountain at a much gentler grade. Certain this was the right way, I started to make my way down the switchback before I decided to save time and slide down a couple shortcuts to scout ahead. I wanted to make sure this was the right direction. Soon enough, I started second guessing myself. Morgan was convinced this route was incorrect, so we went back to the ravine from the way we came.

When we reached the ravine I looked to Morgan and teased her that after all that trouble we had to go back the way from which we had just come. We were on the right path.

We quickly laughed it off.

Given our current mental states, how could we not laugh about our inability to process and remember where all these trails led. We made our way back from a different direction and found ourselves on the switchbacks again, which lead us to the bridge we crossed earlier that morning.

Sleep deprivation makes the memory a bit fuzzy, but as I recall, soon after crossing the bridge we ran into a Death Race Volunteer named Jessica. She radioed back to Joe and tried to stop me, it seemed like she was trying to stir the pot to create more madness.

I kept shushing her off.

At the same time, we ran into fellow Storm Chasers, Mies and Chris along with my crew member, Jennifer. They were on their way out with another racer up the mountain. I asked Jennifer if I could steal her for a bit. She broke-off from the others and came back part of the way to the farm with me. Morgan had a head start and we were less than a mile away now.

What followed was a helpful conversation with Jennifer that was also quite motivational. We hugged it out and she wished me well. It's moments like these that can really help you get through something like the Death Race. A pep talk, pretty girls, hugs, the sun - I was surrounded by positive reinforcement.

Speaking of pep, I added a little bit of it to my shuffle and caught back up with Morgan. With our logs still in tote, we would have to check-in as soon as we returned to the farm. When we finally arrived Joe told us we needed to do burpees as a penalty for taking so long. First, we had to walk over and drop off our logs. A volunteer witnessed the returning of our logs, and we were sent back to Joe.

This was a pretty unique moment of the race. Initially, Margaret Schlachter greeted us. She was recording and live-streaming our check in on Ustream via her female-geared obstacle race blog, Dirt in Your Skirt. We answered some of her questions on the video stream, and then continued to make attempts at moving on to the next task. Joe continued to tell us that not only were we disqualified but he also insisted that we would never finish.

Our minds had been made up and as with all the other attempts to get us to quit, we rushed him to get to the point so we could continue on to our next task. I refused to believe a word he said. I was not out of this race unless I pulled myself out. I dared to start this damn thing, and now had made up my mind, I would finish this thing too.

As it turned out, we were not the only ones suffering from sleep deprivation. Joe gave us our next task and did not at all acknowledge the burpees he threatened us with just a few minutes earlier. What a relief! Thanks, Joe, but mostly thank you, sleep deprivation. At least, that's what I assume caused Joe to forget (or maybe he just decided to be nice...nah...definitely, sleep deprivation). We also got away with only turning in those six logs each and did not have to go back for the other six.

For our next task, we were to trek back-up the hillside to the location where we chopped the wood. No, I am not kidding – we were heading back to virtually the same place we had just come back from. Fair enough. I remember Morgan feeling slightly panicked about our pace, and I stopped her. I told her she needed to STOP worrying and that it was all part of the game. They wanted us to rush and exhaust ourselves. There was no reason to do that, though. We just needed to continue on at a pace that would allow us to finish whatever they threw our way.

Our trek led us back toward the bridge and up the mountain again. We took some shortcuts that led us out back on the road and eased the overall climb. It was interesting to walk so much of the road this time. The last time I had gone this route was when we took the truck up for our weigh in. That felt like so long ago. With the rays of the sun beating down against our skin, the temperature rose, and it became much hotter. Soon our attention shifted to strategizing tactics we could readily implement that would keep us from overheating.

Shade? *Check.*

Water? *Check.*

Gatorade? *Check.*

As we moved up the mountain, which we used for shade, we would switch sides of the road depending on what side provided the most easily accessible canopied areas. Whenever we needed rest, we would hide out under densely covered areas to avoid the Death Race volunteers and staff. Who knew whether or not they would harass you or worse, penalize you? We certainly didn't, so we took precaution.

When we finally arrived at the wood splitting area once again, there were a few volunteers that were hanging out on a picnic bench. Besides them, the rest of this spot had been abandoned. Equipment was just thrown about. An ax, walking sticks, half split wood, buckets, there were so many items just left behind.

We made our way to the table where the volunteers sat. We gave them our names, told them what obstacle we had just completed. They made some marks on their sheets of paper and told us we could head back and move onto the Origami portion. I was surprised to find out that it was just a checkpoint and nothing else.

"Really?" I questioned.

Some of these tasks at the time seemed so silly and tedious to me, but it cracked me up.

Morgan and I about-faced, put our smiles on, and marched off. The key to overcoming adversity is to smile. Just, smile. It'll get you through everything life throws at you.

Now, to the Origami challenge!

We had to head back down the same way we came. Like a shot of caffeine being injected directly into your bloodstream, Morgan and I suddenly found ourselves overcome with a very slap-happy sensation. Our spirits overall were so high. Feeling overly positive about the outcome of this race, I looked to Morgan and said, "You know what, we are going to finish this race. You know why...because *Weeeeeee are the Champions.*"

At that moment I burst out without a care for how awful my singing voice is and began to sing the chorus of the classic Queen hit, *We Are the Champions*. That outburst right there put us in the goofiest mood. We stopped taking ourselves or anything else seriously.

On the descent, we passed a few racers who were headed up, they were moving on to a different challenge. To this day, I am still uncertain what possessed us to start making these comments, but we began to tell tall tales and started messing with other racers that we would see.

We jokingly would say to them we had just finished the race and all we had left to do was make it back to the farm and then we would be the first male and first female finishers to finish at the same time. We just kept making up nonsense about winning and being in first. Some people actually would buy it, if only for a second. Some we admitted to teasing. Others, however, well, we just let them figure it out. It was all in good fun and we were simply making lemonade out of all the lemons we had been given. Truth be told, I thought, we were more likely to be in the last place if anything.

During our return trip, Margaret pulled up and greeted us as she made her way down the road. With her window already rolled down, she looked over at us and began one of the seemingly universal attempts to tell us we were disqualified.

From the beginning of this race and beyond this moment, I lived and breathed by one absolute rule for tackling this Death Race of "Betrayal." That rule was to only listen to Joe and Andy – more importantly we had to know not only when to listen, but what to listen to.

It was tricky, but it left me with a straightforward tactic for handling these situations – don't listen. If they are not Joe and they are not Andy, do not take what they say at face value. Knowing who and what to accept made a world of difference in this race. It was very beneficial having this policy in-place. Ultimately, I would only take direction from the race directors, especially when it came to my status in the event.

Margaret's attempt to break us was simple to shrug off. We felt empowered now. The strength of our pact to finish together grew stronger with every shot taken at us. We wished Margaret farewell and continued to follow the road back down towards Route 100.

Our water supply was beginning to run low, and as if there was a direct link between Morgan and her parents, they suddenly appeared to save the day. As they pulled up, with outstretched arms, they asked us "Do you need some water?"

I was in shock. Literally two minutes prior Morgan and I were discussing our shortage and the need for hydration in this heat. Fortune was in our favor. We kept it brief and quickly they drove off. We had to get moving and we couldn't risk being seen receiving aid. We didn't know whether or not their help would be considered acceptable. Regardless, enough thanks could not be given to Morgan's parents for saving the day.

When we made it to the intersection with Route 100, we were approached by another vehicle, this time it was an SUV with Death Race Volunteers. They told us we could no longer go to the Origami challenge because it had been shut down.

Our response, of course, was, "Where to next?"

This caused them to try to tell us we could not finish and that we would be disqualified.

We didn't accept that and told them, "No, we are continuing on. What's next?"

An unexpected, laughable response followed from the volunteers. They tried to tell us it was a safety issue for us to continue on. My patience grew thin and I snapped back, "I don't know what kind of safety concern there is for you, but we are GOLDEN. We are going to keep going, so please make this easy, tell us what to do next."

They quickly gave in and sent us on our way, "Okay, okay, go see Joe back at the farm."

We took off down Route 100 and ran past the General Store, our spirits were still incredibly high. We said hello to everyone we passed, including a very nice elderly man lounging on his porch. Within ten minutes we found ourselves back at the farm ready to find out what challenges awaited us.

CHAPTER 10

SLEEPYHEAD

"You may encounter many defeats, but you must not be defeated. In fact, it may be necessary to encounter the defeats so you can know who you are, what you can rise from, how you can still come out of it."
~ Maya Angelou

Happily waiting for us at Death Race HQ was Joe De Sena and a few others. It was more than apparent they were surprised with our perseverance. Initially, they didn't want to give us another task but soon enough, they gave in. We just missed participating in the Origami. So, next on their list of challenges required us to head over to the nearby barn. There, a half-full flatbed trailer of hay bales awaited. We were allowed to put our packs down for this challenge. Perfect. My shoulder was feeling some crazy fatigue and this reminded me that I was long overdue for another dose of pain medicine.

Morgan and I immediately set out and each began to sling the 15 required bales of hay. We were required to take the bales from the trailer (however many we could handle at a time) and neatly stack them. Much of the second floor had already been covered from the floorboards to the ceiling rafters by other racers who encountered this obstacle earlier. To play things safe, I started out by taking one bale at a time.

After a couple trips, I decided to attempt speeding things up by bringing two bales. Weight-wise, the task wasn't too difficult, but I quickly found that taking two at a time meant I had to be more cautious during my short trek from the flatbed to the barn. It felt like I had to be too cautious with the finicky hay. Once I had finished carefully moving the two bales at once, I quickly went back to handling one bale at a time. I didn't want to deal with the consequence if a bale fell apart.

Shortly after Morgan and I began transporting the bales of hay into the barn a few more racers arrived and joined us. After their arrival and a few trips to the second floor, I discovered the bales of hay that acted as stairs to the trailer had shifted. I went to step off the trailer, but my foot never found the hay staircase.

TIMMMMMMBERRRRR!!!!

Luckily, I caught myself with the bale of hay I was holding. I moaned and groaned a bit about how uncool it was that the stairs moved, but it was likely an accident. Definitely not betrayal (I think). Regardless, before heading back up for my next bundle I made sure there was a new makeshift staircase in-place and we continued to bring our individual bales. This felt like one of the less-demanding tasks when compared to the rest we dealt with thus far. Upon completion of the task, we gathered our gear and made our way back to uncover our next objective.

Morgan became sidetracked and started to help a few other racers manage their feet before we were able to continue. Many athletes suffered from some of the nastiest foot issues I had ever seen, a result of the hours and hours of them being wet and uncared for. Without proper foot care, some feet end up wholly mangled and sometimes even covered in "trench foot" – it's really quite disgusting.

We are blessed to have people like Morgan in this world. Her heart is so massive, she did not want to let any of our fellow racers suffer (any more than they had to). I watched her go out of her way to help others, even while we were so far behind. Her selflessness was awe-inspiring and showed me an area

I wanted to improve in myself. I found myself genuinely stunned by how much Morgan cared about the other racers.

That is one of the defining aspects in a competition like the Death Race – although everyone competes against one another, there is this sense of camaraderie that manifests and ultimately everyone realizes that we're all in this together. Though we are all in competition, we are also helping one another. When a race is known for its 80% (or higher) failure rate, it is easy for the participants to band together to try to defeat those odds.

As Morgan finished tending to a racer's foot, I encouraged her to speed things up so we could continue on to the next part of the race. Her selflessness and desire to help other racers was admirable, but the reality of our situation was that we were many, many hours behind. At that moment, I feared we would jeopardize our status if we were to fall even further behind. I didn't want to end up finding ourselves so far behind that we couldn't recover, again.

Nevertheless, I was proud to be teamed-up with Morgan. We made our short trek back from the hay bales and checked-in with our overlords. Our next task involved carrying a bag of cement mix up to the top of the mountain. Joe explained that not only were we disqualified but he further insisted that we would never finish. If we chose to go on, we would be unofficially in the race.

We would not be deterred.

Our minds were made up. As with all the other attempts to get us to quit, we just rushed him to get to the point. All we wanted was for Joe to move us on to the next obstacle we needed to best. Joe didn't let up though; he kept on about how we could never finish, *officially*.

I stood resolute, refusing to believe a word he said.

The back-and-forth went on for a short while. We asked Joe if we could have our cement bags and move along. All Morgan and I wanted was to continue. Surprisingly, we were informed there were no cement bags for us and we were instructed to just move on. I still didn't understand how this happened and would have loved to take on that challenge. Little did I know that years later my wish would come true.

It still irks me that we were brushed off from this challenge. Sure, my shoulder was dead, but the endorphins were firing at full force and I am confident that my sheer determination and persistence in that moment alone would have been enough to get us to the top of that mountain with whatever weight they gave us.

Just before we departed for the next challenge, I spoke with my crew member, Jennifer, about coming with for the next task. I would have loved to have a little extra support with someone to talk to. She just returned from a hike herself so it was no surprise she would want some rest. There were no hard feelings but it was a little unfortunate that we weren't syncing up.

Fortunately, I had met a formidable partner to run with me. I knew it would be all right moving forward. As we attempted to head-out, we found ourselves blocked-off by one of the animal pens. Instead of taking the street back like we were instructed to, we used this opportunity to just go back up the trail we had used every other time.

Once we got back on-track, the next ascent back up the mountain was one of the toughest. Morgan and I were both becoming extremely delusional. I recall growing hyper-aware in the moment of the rambling and nonsensical chatter that I was spewing forth. I had a hard time understanding half the words that came out of my mouth. Sleep deprivation was unquestionably taking its toll on us and the results were hysterical.

Times like these would be pure comedic gold if caught on camera and recorded! We couldn't continue on without putting ourselves at risk. It had finally reached a point where it was out of necessity that we needed to take a break to close our eyes. Our levels of sleep deprivation were growing ever more uglier in this environment. People say being sleep deprived is more disorientating than being drunk, and with the rambling and stumbling I experienced – that assertion was more than accurate.

So for our safety, we took a nap.

People often wonder, *how in the holy hell did they take a nap out on the mountain in the middle of a trail?*

Well, it's quite simple, really – we dropped our packs and I took out my iPhone and set the alarm for ten minutes.

Voilà!

Naptime.

The most challenging part of naptime was the fear of other racers seeing us. After that fear came the dismay of some unknown animal discovering our location or worse, coming after us. My senses were on high alert. The wind blowing would freak me out and wake me up within two minutes of closing my eyes. We never actually slept, but shutting our eyes for those few minutes was what we needed to push through and continue.

During our trek through the mountain, we saw a lot of printouts of the same images from the hints we saw before race start. At first, I didn't think much of it. However, as we kept seeing more printouts, I started to wonder if this was the last obstacle coming up. We came to a clearing and out of nowhere came Morgan's mother and father running to us. They came from nearby where the next challenge took place. Beyond seeing their daughter again, there was a purpose to them coming toward us with such haste. It turned out they had done some recon work and had intel for us.

Sweeeet.

They shared with us two of the questions and answers being asked as part of the next challenge.

Q. What sense is most connected to memory?

A. Smell

Q. Which athlete does the most squats during their sport?

A. Catcher

Very odd questions, I thought. Morgan's parents gave us a rundown of the upcoming challenge and explained to us that they were not allowed to help Morgan, but they could help me. At the time, I didn't understand why, but that common reminder that this was the Death Race meant one thing – you just gotta go with it.

Morgan and I made our way over to the challenge, and Jack began to explain to us the most intense obstacle we would face yet.

Mark was there. It was good to see him smiling and supporting the rest of us who were still in it.

When the task was first presented to us, I underestimated the difficulty of the challenge. To finish this obstacle, we were to perform a log roll, lying on your side and rolling your body... yes, like a log, through a quarter mile loop. At the halfway point a bucket was strategically placed.

What was inside the bucket? I thought.

The answer was far more unpleasant than I could have imagined.

Rotting intestines and other internal organs from a bull that had been left out in the hot scorching sun for the past two months. Gross. And of course, we were to stir the contents of said bucket ten times during each lap of the log rolling course by using a broken branch they left for us to use in the bucket.

Six laps. That's how many times we were expected to roll around this quarter mile loop and stir this bucket of vile content. Joy.

CHAPTER 11

NEVER QUIT, NEVER SURRENDER

"Do, or do not. There is no try." ~ Yoda

We were back at Riverside Farm for the last challenge. For starters, you needed to have a ticket if you wanted to "ride". If you did not have a ticket you could earn one by doing 120 push-ups. Thanks to a tip from Morgan's parents, I quickly grabbed a notecard out of my bag. I tore the card in half and wrote "ticket" on both cards. Thinking I was clever, I told them, "Of course I bought the tickets for our first date."

And just like that, we gained our "admission" to the main event.

Jack, the Administrator of this event, further instructed us that at the end of each lap we had to answer a question of his choosing. A correct answer made the lap count, a wrong answer meant you were re-rolling an entire lap. Now it all made sense why Morgan's parents wanted us to know the answers to those questions. Still, even prepared with that knowledge, this made for a very interesting obstacle. We only knew two of the however many questions Jack had prepared.

Before setting off on our first lap, I made some adjustments to my gear. Additionally, we were able to set aside our bags, which was a very welcome relief. Jack made sure to insist countless times about the toxicity of the contents of the bucket. I really had no clue what we were up against. Out of fear of anything being too poisonous on the course I took every possible precaution. From the depths of my pack, I took out my long sleeve compression shirt. For leg coverage, I was already equipped with long compression socks. In addition to those layers, I put on a pair of construction gloves and I made myself a bandit-style face mask from my bandana.

Finally, I was ready to rock. Jack made a comment that I was the first to think of covering my face and that it was probably a brilliant idea.

Overconfidence in my abilities led to a brutal test of everything I had to give. In large part, because of my background in gymnastics, I assumed I was capable of handling more speed. I threw myself into the fastest log roll I have ever performed. For some reason, I thought to myself that maybe, just maybe, I had a chance to pass some people up for once. My competitive edge was kicking in during the final hours. The effort was probably futile, but being competitive is one of those things in which you either are, or are not.

That day, I was.

Up to this point, the average time for completing a single lap was somewhere around 25-30 minutes. I knew I could obliterate that time at the pace I was going. Now, I am not one hundred percent positive exactly how fast I finished the first lap, but the looks I was given when I completed it said it all.

I dominated it.

It was somewhere under fifteen minutes. It's not like they were *not* timing us.

When I finished the first lap, Jack asked me the "smell" question. Of course, I answered correctly and the other racers who finished beside me had the option to take the gamble and go with my answer. They all chose to gamble. We were congratulated for a correct answer and my first lap was marked on a whiteboard next to my name.

The only trying parts about that first lap were the few pinecones we had to avoid while rolling through some mulch and stirring the bucket of guts — which was disgusting.

I waited for Morgan before starting the second lap. As soon as she was ready we went back for more. My second lap would be a huge reality check for me. About halfway through the lap, I started to feel nauseous.

Was it the rolling?

Was it the smell?

It didn't matter...I had to get up and, and....BLARGHHH.

That was vomit episode number one. Morgan's dad, who was following alongside us, passed me some water. I sucked it down and continued. Shortly after stirring the bucket I met Captain Vomit, again. It felt awful. Morgan's parents continued to encourage me to persist.

I correctly answered the question about smell again and prepared myself for the next lap.

Facing the third lap wasn't too bad, but I definitely slowed down more each round. Throughout that lap, Morgan's parents gave me water and Gatorade. They were the best supporters I could have out there. It was so incredibly kind of them to help me out.

Thankfully during the third lap, I only found it necessary to puke once. Regardless of the vomiting, Morgan and I were still in high spirits. Luckily for her, she didn't have the recurring need to spew her guts out. Everyone participating would randomly sing any and every song you could think of that had a verse about rolling, despite how much vomit we now rolled through.

When I got back to Jack, I once again answered the question about smell. As it turned out, Jack was rotating between just a few questions. The smell one being the most frequent, of course. After the fourth lap, which I thankfully completed puke-free, I needed to just lie down for a second.

Morgan's mother, Dian, agreed to give me five minutes. She made sure to get me back up to keep going. Five minutes was not enough. Suddenly, I was feeling awful.

I shot up from where I laid and realized I needed to go take care of business in the woods. This was one of the most awkward moments of my life. At the time it was out of necessity with a touch of absent-mindedness on top. I knew Morgan had baby wipes but completely forgot to grab them before heading out into the woods. I had no time to think and I ran off into the woods.

Before I even had a chance to pull my pants down, I found myself puking again! Once all the toxins were out, I turned around and dropped trou.

Without baby wipes.

Oh, no!

It was bad. I needed wipes. I couldn't believe I was going to do this.

"Morgan!!!" I shouted.

"I need baby wipes."

Poor girl. However, these were desperate times. Morgan arrived quickly and handed me a couple wipes and ran off. I never imagined I would find myself so vulnerable. I had no time to even think about that at the time. This was not the time to be shy, and thankfully Morgan was a team player.

The moments following my bathroom break were harsh. My body began to give up on me. It began to shut-down. It felt like it was failing me. Snot clogged my nose and yet it also poured out all simultaneously.

Suddenly, I found myself shivering uncontrollably. The entirety of my body shook. Instead of going back to where the rest of the Death Racers were continuing to roll around in each others vomit, I returned to the clearing where we saw Morgan's parents just before walking up to it.

I found a flat spot and I curled up in a ball and tried to get my shit back together.

I thought to myself, *What is happening to me?*

After expelling fluids from every orifice, I had utterly depleted myself of all the calories and water. But it didn't matter.

I refused to give in.

Morgan came to my aid and made a fire. Her mother cut up what I was told were a pair of Morgan's grandfather's socks, to create sleeves. She covered the only uncovered part of my body, my knees. Morgan's father, Derek, provided me with a vest to increase my body temperature and bring me some relief in the form of warmth.

With snot spewing out of my nose and, of course, now after being shown all this love from strangers, came a waterfall of tears – uncontrollable, heartfelt tears. It was as though every body part that had a releasable fluid wanted to join in on the fun.

I stumbled to find my words, "I. Am. Not. Giving. Up. I have come too damn far to quit this damn race."

Morgan felt differently.

She couldn't stand seeing me like this and thought maybe we should call it quits.

"Quit?"

"Hell, no! Not now. We've come too far."

I told her it wasn't an option. We had to finish. We had a pact.

My Warrior's Ethos dog tag pressed against my chest.

A reminder:

I will always place the mission first.

I will never accept defeat.

I will never quit.

I will never leave a fallen comrade.

In that moment, I remembered how great I felt when Todd Sedlak presented me those tags just six months earlier. It was at my 26th birthday, which was unforgettable. I was thankful for having met Todd and for all that I had learned from him in that short time. His tips and tricks played a significant role in my success.

From the location of the Death Race "rollercoaster" (the way the challenge induced us to vomit, it seemed like a fitting name) another racer, Stacie, emerged. Stacie dropped earlier but stuck around to help others throughout the event. She came over to check on me. I remember upon seeing her, the first thing I asked of her was for a hug. It was immensely comforting, among the most comforting hugs I have experienced. Sometimes, all you need is love – and the love that comes from a hug can go a long way.

Stacie and Morgan spent time cheering me up and they switched over to encouraging me and telling me that I was awesome for making it this far. The whole group helped bring me back to life. They revitalized me with food, water, fire, and clothing. It's all about the essentials. The simple things in life. This race reminded me of what is important. Being kind to one another was the best thing this race brought out of others.

Before heading back out, Morgan wanted to lie down to get some rest. I was anxious to get back out there, but figured, what was another couple of minutes after racing for over 50 something hours. Morgan laid herself down in front of me by the fire. I cuddled up next to her. Sharing our body warmth was pleasant but I refused to rest for long. Within less than ten minutes I woke Morgan up. It was time to finish what we started. I felt invigorated. After facing what felt like something I wouldn't be able to rebound from, to being back to my peppy-self, was nothing short of unbelievable, especially to myself. Thanks to the help of these selfless humans, I had a new found determination to conquer this infernal race.

While I vomited and shat my brains out, Morgan had pulled

off an extra lap, which left her with only one lap to go while I still had two. She insisted that she would complete both with me, regardless of what I told her. I was impressed by her selflessness – it seemed to know no bounds. No matter how awful and unpleasant another lap was, Morgan was determined to see that we both finished. For this, I am forever grateful.

By the time we reported back to Jack for the last laps, the sun had set. Everywhere we looked was washed in shades of black. There was very little light besides the occasionally blinding starburst of light from everyone's headlamps. The darkness would play to our advantage for the next two laps. After clocking in my fifth lap and Morgan's sixth, she revealed her plan to Jack about doing another lap with me. He was stunned a racer would voluntarily do another lap of misery just to help someone else to finish. He was so impressed that he radioed the news to Joe and Andy. It would seem this took them both off-guard. With the guidance of Morgan's father, Morgan and I set out on my final lap together.

We finished the lap at a nice pace and answered the final question. One last attempt to trigger our sense of smell. You're a sick man, Jack. What Jack orchestrated here is quite awful. By repeatedly asking this question to many a sleep-deprived racer going through many, many hours of Hell, Jack had, in essence, programmed the smell of guts into our collective memory. It seemed from my perspective in the race, to be the only question he asked. Too bad his question had a 100% failure rate on us. Thankfully, everyone answered that question correct, everytime.

After finishing the final lap, Jack requested for us to let him know when we had our gear and we were ready to continue. We didn't need long to gather our belongings as everything was ready to go, right where we left it.

"Where to next Jack? We're ready," we said.

When Jack radioed Joe he received an unexpected response. Previously, Joe had been directing racers to go meet at the top of the mountain, but this time he told Jack to hold us there.

Hold us here? Are we really unable to finish? Are we really unofficial?

Concern briefly overwhelmed me.

And so we did all we could do – we waited. Other racers were continually coming through the rolling section. Answering that same question to tie that smell to the racers' memory over and over.

After what seemed like an eternity of waiting we spotted Andy as he approached us. At first, it seemed as though he lurked in the darkness, but I quickly noticed he was in very high spirits. Andy went around asking a few racers how they were doing. He gathered an idea of everyone's thoughts and feelings regarding the rolling challenge.

When Andy came up to us and asked us how we felt about it, he looked over to Jack and confirmed that we had finished our laps. Jack made sure to point out how Morgan was the only racer to voluntarily complete seven total laps. Andy was pumped. He loved it and he looked at both of us and said six words.

Six words that meant more to me than, well, words could ever possibly describe.

"Congratulations, you finished the Death Race."

WHAT?!

"No way!" we shouted.

We were completely shocked.

We did it.

We finished.

We finished the Death Race.

We finished the Death Race.

WE. FINISHED. THE. DEATH. RACE!

Overcome by excitement, we quickly calmed ourselves to listen to the last of his instructions. All we needed to do was walk across the field and over to the pool house to claim our trophy.

Really?! I thought.

I couldn't believe it.

Is this real life?!

Death Race: Vanquished

We made our way over to the small shack. We were greeted by Margaret and Chris. They had relocated the HQ that was set up down at Amee Farm to this new location near Riverside Farm. The red LED lights of the clock displayed over 58 hours. Margaret didn't know what our actual status was, but she questioned it and told us we had to await confirmation.

Seriously?!

The mind games never ended! Andy came in and confirmed it. In his delusional state he congratulated us and he awarded Morgan as the second place female. Obviously after all we had gone through we were completely taken by surprise, we were shocked but also completely pumped. This was tremendous news, but our initial shock was more than warranted, after all we were declared unofficial all throughout the second half of the event.

As you would imagine, we eventually discovered Andy's sleep deprivation got the best of him. Like all of us who raced, sleep escaped our race director. The reality was fellow Illinoisan (at the the time), Amelia Boone, placed second. In mine and Morgan's case, we simply finished the race. Unofficially.

Although a few challenges were incomplete, we still fought through everything we were told to. We conquered every obstacle presented. We went from each destination we were told to the next.

We battled through feelings of defeat.

We overcame the trials of the human mind's ability to persevere, even when all odds were against us. Morgan and I went through the transformation from being mere acquaintances to being able to trust and rely on each other in moments that would crush most people and swallow them whole. The quest to finish the Death Race had come to an end.

We completed the Death Race.

I finished the Death Race.

Sure, the Death Race is an individuals event but having someone to partner up with for the race, especially someone as wonderful, uplifting, and positive as Morgan, that alone played a major part in my finish. There is just no better secret weapon. The power of human camaraderie can conquer anything.

Morgan's parents snapped a photo of our finish.

We did it.

I did it.

I didn't think I could ever be happier than that moment...(I was wrong). The two of us hung-out for a while and saw the top two male finishers come in. These guys had finished every single task that was prescribed by the race organizers. Many of those tasks I never got a chance to face because of the whole tire fiasco, that was the difference between earning an unofficial finish that year, or being like these guys and earning the glorified "official" finish.

In first place was Olof Dallner, a fellow friend I met through the Storm Chasers Spartan group and in second place, Junyong Pak. They had the extra task of summiting the mountain once again. Those two guys are some of the most incredible athletes I've ever had the pleasure of racing alongside. How the race organizers managed to track everything seemed mind-boggling to me at the time but I just trusted they knew who earned what.

Margaret was walking around with her iPhone live streaming the event before live streaming was the cool thing to do. Using a service called Ustream, she live-streamed the reactions of racers after finishing. While she was streaming the event, I was on the phone with my dad and I thought it was so neat that he could tune in. Thankfully my father was able to log-on, and he watched me say hello to him after finishing. Sometimes, technology is magical. Being able to share that moment with my dad, it was the icing on the cake.

Morgan's parents asked me where I was headed. Since I had never booked a hotel, there seemed to be no need to since the race was expected to conclude Monday, I had no clue. It was now Monday. Just after midnight. They offered the only thing they could, which was more than I needed, a hardwood floor inside a hotel. We went back to the Trailside Inn. Morgan showered first, then I had my turn. I did my best to clean off the three days of stench. Once we were both clean we threw on our Death Race hoodies, and we all shared a glass of wine. I took a look at how gnarly my feet were and snapped a great photo. Before I passed out, I made plans to meet up with Mark in the early morning.

The next morning Morgan's parents dropped me off by Mark back at Amee Farm. He had already gotten most of my things packed for me. We said our goodbyes and that was it.

The Death Race was over.

It ended so fast. Which is funny because at times during the event it felt that the misery and punishment would never pass.

But the memories would last a lifetime and now they will last even longer. Mark drove us back to his place in New Hampshire from Vermont. After another shower, we shared a few beers while we iced our poor, tattered feet and soon enough it was time to head to the airport. Mark dropped me off and we hugged it out. I took the next flight back to Chicago.

I did it.

I was a Death Race finisher, unofficially. The **Year of Betrayal**... vanquished, unofficially.

But this wouldn't be the end of it.

CHAPTER 12

THE MONTHS AFTER DEATH

"True freedom is impossible without a mind made free by discipline."
~ Mortimer J. Adler

The next few months after having "unofficially" finished the Death Race, I realized that my fight was not over. Initially, I knew I would have to go through with having surgery on my torn shoulder before I could continue competing in more of these obstacle racing and endurance racing-style events.

It was a difficult decision to make, but it was something I had decided during the event. After suffering so much pain performing numerous carrying tasks at the race, it was time to get the one-inch labrum tear repaired. It wasn't enough to merely have the Courage to finish the first event. I needed to have the Power to do every challenge so that I could become an official finisher. *Unofficial* just was not enough. I spent many nights waking cold and drenched, soaked in sweat with the fleeting thoughts racing through my head – that I was still out there, on the mountain, trying to finish the Death Race.

I had unfinished business. My dance with the Death Race had not come to a close. However, I had a shoulder to fix first.

I did what any dedicated athlete would, I went and found the best surgeon I could. Luckily for me, I found one of the best right there in my hometown of Chicago. Dr. Mark Bowen, with a resume including serving as the Team Physician for the Chicago Bears, and also acting as Team Physician to the Chicago Blackhawks, Chicago Cubs, New York Giants, and the Big Ten Conference, was a specialist in shoulders and knees. In my mind, if Dr. Bowen had the skills and techniques that enabled these big-time professional athletes to get back to competition after suffering similar types of awful muscle tears, I was confident he could do the same for me.

It's never just the surgeon though, it's the PT, physical therapy, too. Without the proper physical therapy and diligence regarding the corrective exercises to heal and strengthen the affected area, the surgery becomes less effective.

After shoulder surgery, I was in a tremendous amount of pain for weeks. I had a prescription to numb the pain but avoided using it as much as possible. I didn't want to touch that stuff again after having felt how much of a grip it can have on you.

Ten months prior to surgery I had become addicted to the relief I got from those painkillers. Every night I would take two. Then when it was time for surgery, I had to stop taking the pills. It was difficult. I couldn't believe it but I was afraid to come off the pills. I even expressed how fearful I was of not having those pills to mask my pain to my doctor. He told me I had to stop taking them for a month before surgery if I wanted any pain relief when he cut me up and stitched me back together. I obliged. It was shockingly difficult. Once I realized this, I came to the conclusion that I would minimize my use of opioid painkillers. The risk of addiction was already far too high.

While I had the pills available after my surgery, I minimized my use of them, and only took them in the early stages of recovery. Icing my shoulder became my favorite activity of the day. It felt so good every time I iced my shoulder that I would ice up to five times a day.

At first, I worked from home, but eventually I had to return to work and find a ride to get me there and back. At that point, I was in a sling and was not allowed to move my elbow away from my side. My angle had to be, as my doctor put it, "Velcroed to your side." I was very protective of my shoulder and arm for the entire duration of my gimp-status.

Six weeks after surgery I started my road to recovery at Athletico in Bloomingdale, Illinois under the guidance of an exceptionally well trained Physical Therapist by the name of Alysha. She helped me focus to regain all that I had lost. When I arrived at my first session, I had not moved my shoulder much at all. The exception being all the arm circle pendulums I did on a daily basis per Dr. Bowen's guidance.

I could barely lift my arm that first session. The muscle was so tender and weak from having my labrum repaired and reattached to the bone. With my extremely limited range of motion I felt powerless and pathetic. I was barely able to put my hoodie on and taking it off was even worse.

Alysha and I went straight to work with implementing a regimen of exercises and stretches that built on one another. Every week or two my therapy would evolve. The progression included more exercises, increased range of motion, isometrics, heavier weight, higher resistance – it was wonderful. Everyday activities became easier. Eating, for instance, was simple again. Reaching for something in the cabinet, brushing my teeth, all the daily actions that most people take for granted became increasingly more doable. The chance to increase my strength and return to racing inched closer, and I became hungry to race. After sitting on the sidelines and watching the Winter Death Race play-out, I felt encouraged and even more eager to get my shoulder healed.

My discipline and dedication to doing my physical therapy diligently paid off. I was a few weeks ahead of schedule in the healing process. The official day for me to start to add more strength exercises was February 22, 2013 and I was scheduled to conclude all of my prescribed therapy on March 14th.

At the time, I was newly unemployed from a round of layoffs and my insurance only lasted through the last week of February. I couldn't let that stop my progress. So, starting

March 1st, I switched to at home therapy under the guidance of my mother who was a professional bodybuilder and personal trainer, and who had enough background in physical therapy and training to help me continue from where Alysha left off.

Alysha left us with a plan to execute, and she even took the time to see me once more a few weeks later for a follow-up consultation to make sure I was on the right path.

***

The process of undergoing this surgery and the recovery involved was one of my life's most challenging obstacles to overcome. I had to dig deep to overcome bouts of depression from the lack of exercise and movement.

On one side of the coin, I found myself happy, but as humans we tend to remember the good and forget the bad. Looking back from a more realistic perspective reveals that my recovery could be represented by a fairly typical ECG graph, with repeating sets of high highs and low lows followed by a lot of steady segments. Recovery required a lot of discipline and determination. It was a tough battle at times but it was so much better than the pain and discomfort I had dealt with prior to surgery, and it only got better with each passing day.

When you are injured, it's like you are being torn away from all of the things that bring you happiness, and for a period of time you find you have to give up the thing you love most. Even if it is only temporarily, it is quite daunting, especially mentally. It takes a lot of courage and power to overcome the mental and physical struggle you must endure to get back to being you. I found I had to constantly remind myself, "this is where I am now and it's okay to be where I am as long as I am working toward my goal," which I was, every day.

In many ways the months of recovery were quite interesting. I went from not leaving my house due to doctors orders not to drive, to having the freedom to go anywhere and everywhere. There were a lot of milestones I hit during my recovery and each one made me incredibly appreciative of my ability to move my body.

After three weeks of doing diligent at-home recovery, I went back to see Alysha. I had something I wanted to show her. When I walked in, I glowed, I had been working hard at rebuilding the strength in my shoulder, and I recently hit a new milestone, I was able to do a pull-up. A couple in a row in fact!

With this knowledge in the back of my mind, I told Alysha, "I can do a pull-up."

She responded, "There's no way."

I laughed and said, "Just watch."

I jumped up on the pull-up bar and did not one, not two, not three or four, but five! I did five full-extension pull-ups four months post-op. Even I was impressed, I knew I could do at least two when I jumped up. I wanted to impress my Physical Therapist, after all, it was her hard work that got me there. I wanted her to see how much that work had paid off. She did a few tests and told me that I apparently had things figured out, I was told to play it smart, take it slowly, but was given the go-ahead to begin training again.

When I asked if I could do the Death Race that was about 80 days away, she laughed and suggested we evaluate how well I was doing as the race got closer.

A month later, I tagged along with some friends for the Spartan Super in Vegas. At the race venue I met up with some of my friends from Team SISU and Team Tire. During the race I discovered the most difficult obstacle for me at this stage of recovery was the bucket carry. I couldn't do it, yet. It was a bit concerning with the 2013 Death Race a mere 60 days away, but all I could do was keep working on myself, training, recovering, rehabilitating, and doing everything it took, simply improving one day after the other.

Two months later, it was time to return to the battlefield.

Entering my second year of Death Racing, I was playing for keeps, after all this was the **Year of the Gambler.**

Had I developed enough power to survive? Only time would tell.

YEAR 2
POWER

"You have power over your mind — not outside events. Realize this, and you will find strength"

~Marcus Aurelius

CHAPTER 13

JET-SETTER

"Optimism is the faith that leads to achievement. Nothing can be done without hope and confidence." ~ Helen Keller

The Week of June 17, 2013

—

A week before the 2013 Death Race, I attended a training camp that was designed as the premier training for Spartan Race and Obstacle Race related programming. The program, originally named Spartan Group X Training at that time, which has since evolved into SpartanSGX, made for an educationally-rewarding and memorable trip to California.

On this trip I seized a chance to take in a lot of what California has to offer. I started off in San Diego and made my way up the Pacific Coast to San Luis Obispo where I stayed for a few days before heading back down the coast. At the time, San Luis Obispo, or SLO as it's referred to by locals, was ranked the happiest city in the United States; pretty cool place to be if you ask me. To top it all off, I had a unique opportunity to participate in the competitive heat of a race that, to this day, is the most obstacle-dense race to hit the circuit.

In my humble opinion, this race came the closest that any company has to producing and designing an Olympic-worthy race format for the sport of obstacle course racing. Alpha Warrior, as it was called, was a course that clocked in just under one-mile but in that short distance managed to cram in over 48 obstacles. This incredibly challenging obstacle race was erected in the parking lot of the San Diego Chargers.

Returning home after the trip, I was beyond ecstatic about what transpired and what lay ahead. But, as I flew back from San Diego the Monday night before the Death Race I suddenly felt the nerves begin to trigger and I could feel a slight bit of anxiety building within my body. Before leaving to California, I pre-prepared and had already packed most of the necessities for the Death Race, so that when I returned I only had a few things I would gather. In the past year, I learned to over-prepare. The more prepared I was for the unexpected, the more power I would have to overcome any obstacles thrown my way, or so I thought.

My flight from San Diego to Chicago's O'Hare International Airport arrived at 11:59 PM on Monday. I had to fly out to Manchester, New Hampshire on Wednesday at 6:00 AM from O'Hare, arriving 1:34 PM in Cleveland for a layover and a perfect place for naptime. Everything leading up to this Death Race was cutting things close. I thought I did enough to prepare ahead of time, but when it came down to it, packing was a nightmare.

Luckily for me, my pops – my father and the man who has always been there for me in everything I do – took the time while I was traveling to find someone to have my beloved Fiskars x27 Axe sharpened.

On Tuesday, I spent the day gathering my gear and had to go on a shopping frenzy to get some last minute necessities. All of the last minute scrambling around evoked a sense that the race had already begun. Pure enjoyment and happy smiles were in full effect even though my mind raced faster than a Ferrari on the Autobahn. Although at times I felt like I was bound to forget all the essentials in my constant haste, nothing could wipe that massive grin off my face. I kept reminding myself that 90% of what I needed was packed and this last 10% could not be prepared for. This was just the nature of this event. Releasing last minute gear lists and changes to the gear list were all a part of what made this event such an utter mindfuck.

When I arrived in Manchester, New Hampshire Mark Webb picked me up from the airport and we did even more shopping. The two of us still needed food and a few other oddities for the race such as: grass seed, hydration in the form of gallons of water and Pedialyte, a hand shovel, a compression sack, and some Colgate Wisps – a secret weapon for multi-day adventures – and all the other stuff you don't want to have to fly with when trying to minimize luggage weight.

While I was traveling, I thought about how far I had come since the year prior. Just a year ago, I was six months into suffering a one-inch labrum tear to my left shoulder. Now, I was seven months post-op, and I was feeling better than ever. Even I was impressed with how much strength and power I was able to develop in such a short amount of time – muscle memory, I suppose.

This year would be a test of my power – a test of how far I had come since overcoming all the trials of the year prior. I learned to overcome my fear of the unknown and gained the courage to start and finish something that the old version of myself would have no business doing. The previous year, I felt like I possessed enough strength to get by, but the reality is I was also competing under the influence of strong pain-inhibiting narcotics to deal with my torn shoulder.

The difficult truth was for a brief period of time I was actually hooked on them.

In the months leading up to my surgery to repair the torn labrum in my left shoulder I went through withdrawals as I weaned myself off the prescription to Norco.

After surgery I tried hard not to rely on the painkillers to get through the recovery. I was thankful to be entering this race entirely clean of those addictive painkillers. The days leading up to my second dance with Death, I realized that I hadn't taken Norco in months – and, let me tell you, it felt really good.

Much like the year prior, Mark and I were headed to the Death Race, together. We met in Manchester, New Hampshire where Mark resides full-time. Connecting with Mark and heading over to Vermont became a fun tradition over the years and it is one that I still treasure.

When it came down to it, one of my favorite things about making the excursion out to Vermont to compete in this *Sufferfest* where it was me against me had absolutely nothing to do with me at all. My favorite thing was seeing, being, and racing among some of the bravest, most courageous and powerful people I have ever met.

I'm thankful to be able to call so many of these seekers of personal growth my friends. In this tight-knit community there are all these genuinely inspiring individuals and I was able to surround myself with their energy, ambition, and esteem, which brought tremendous happiness into my life.

When Mark and I arrived near the race venue we headed down the road where we checked into the Hillside Inn located in Killington, Vermont just ten minutes from Pittsfield, Vermont where the race venue was located.

The evening before the race we ventured a bit closer to Pittsfield to meet up with our close group of Death Race friends to enjoy what became another sort of tradition for us Death Racers. Whether it was the Summer Death Race or the Winter Death Race, Team SISU always rented out this house near the venue. Every year, the night before the race, we would host a "Last Supper" of sorts. It was a great place to hypothesize about the event, discuss tactics, gear, and all the ins and outs of why we do what we do.

Earlier that year I attended another one of these "Last Supper" dinners at the Winter Death Race. At that time, I was still in an arm sling and I hadn't even begun my post-op physical therapy yet. Fast-forward five months and here I was ready to race. However, this time it was much more enjoyable especially since I didn't have to constantly protect my shoulder.

After dinner, Mark and I headed back for an early night at the hotel. We needed to be at registration by 9:00 AM at the latest on Friday morning. We discussed it back-and-forth and eventually decided that we would head out to try to drop our gear at Amee Farm and then head to the Original General Store to grab a hearty breakfast.

When we pulled up at Amee Farm we were told we were not allowed to park there for our gear drop. In the distance, we could see Amelie Boone doing the same exact thing that Mark and I just requested to do. It mildly irked me while I tried to enjoy breakfast. For whatever reason, I kept breakfast simple and stuck to a bowl of granola, yogurt, and fruit.

After spending some time fueling ourselves and reconnecting with other racers, Mark and I decided to try giving it another go at Amee Farm. This time we succeeded. We showed the "parking security" volunteer the email pointing out that we could indeed drop our gear anytime after 5:00 AM at Amee Farm and with that email in front of him he agreed to allow us to proceed.

While we unpacked a staff member approached us – and just like that, the mind games began. This staff member kept going on and on that we were incredibly late for registration and that we would never make it in time to start. Both Mark and I kept doing what we needed to unload his vehicle and secure our location in the gear tent. We refused to let his incessant "You'll never make it" talk distract or disturb us. By now, having participated and witnessed a few Death Races first hand, I was starting to understand how all of it worked and it started to crack me up how much effort the staff and volunteers would put into convincing a racer to drop or quit.

Once everything was unloaded, it was off to Riverside Farm to park Mark's vehicle and drop-off our identification and one other item deemed valuable. Holding these items was their method of keeping track of everyone. No one was going to leave without these essential life items. I entrusted them with my expired DePaul Student ID and my much more valuable Driver's License, so they had at least one thing I would want to get back.

When we pulled up, we parked next to a group of fellow Midwesterners, the Corn Fed Spartans, who were some of my teammates and support crew. TJ Nomeland looked ready to go, but uncertainty about when to start showed in his eyes. There's this game that exists where the sooner you show up, the more work you find yourself subjected to. Knowing this, we all waited until nearly 8:30 AM to register, knowing from the email that it was from 6:00 AM until 9:00 AM.

Now that I was a veteran I had accrued knowledge about how things worked, it's the kind of knowledge that first-timers are usually not privy to. The sooner you show up at the Death Race, the sooner you go to work, and that work doesn't stop until the Race Directors say you finished the Death Race or you pull yourself from the course. The more you do during the Death Race, the sooner and more likely you are to overwork yourself and find yourself with a DNF, or a Did Not Finish status. It's just the fact of this race. That's the Death Race. There is a balance to find in playing the Death Race game.

After all, this was the **Year of the Gambler**.

And all of us were gambling by making it this far. Up until the race I was uncertain how gambling would tie into the race, but it was all starting to make sense. Everything you do in the race, the choices you make, the food you eat, the shoes you wear, it's all a gamble.

The race itself was a gamble.

Completing a challenge and knowing you completed it – that's a gamble. We were gambling with when to register and when we would choose to begin the race.

We decided we would start at 9:00 AM. The first place we got sent to was Andy's new home as he had just moved from Illinois to Vermont. On the way, we had a checkpoint that involved using our hand snips to trim some foliage along the trailside. Right off the bat, typical Death Race landscaping work would be the first task. If you ask me, after all these years, it's still just as hilarious as it was then. By registering for this race we essentially paid to do trail work. It's an impressive business model for sure, but that's an entirely different book to write.

Back to the trail work, I tried to get my snips out, but somehow while I went to pull them out of my bag, I misplaced them. For about five minutes I searched trying to find them. Suddenly, everyone was being sent onward to Andy's just as I clipped my first branch. Relieved to have found my snips, I quickly packed my stuff up and moved on. I tried to stay hyper-aware of everything that was happening within my immediate bubble – I figured that was all that mattered. I felt it in my gut, within a few more minutes we'd be kicking off this dangerous, twisted, challenging race.

"Am I ready?" I asked myself.

"Absolutely," I told myself. *"You've got this. No thoughts, no worries, just do whatever task they ask, and move on to the next challenge, it's just one foot in front of the other. One challenge at a time. You've got this. You can do this. Be a robot."*

The **Year of the Gambler** had finally begun. The time to test my post-op power was here at last.

CHAPTER 14

STAIRWAY TO HEAVEN

"What you do makes a difference, and you have to decide what kind of difference you want to make." - Jane Goodall

As I made my way over to Andy's residence, I could feel the muddy terrain beneath the grip of the Inov-8 Roclite 285 model of trail shoes. It was slick and challenging, but the shoes kept my feet planted and stable despite the unpleasant footing. The path that led to Andy's was relatively short and straightforward to navigate. As we arrived, we came to a sudden halt. It was time for a gear check by none other then the children of the race directors.

It is pretty hysterical how often they would involve their kids in playing games with the racers. And, as a matter of fact, the kids were pretty damn good at it, too. I hopped out of the line and went off to the side for a brief moment. Somehow, that action was interpreted as me "cutting" the line when in actuality all I had intended was to open my ruck to locate my index card. You see, that card had everything I packed written on it along with the specific gear from the required gear list. I quickly showed the three items requested to be seen by the children and then I packed my gear up – ready for whatever hell would await.

In the front of his home, Andy was wandering around the

various groups of racers. He greeted the veterans with a certain enthusiasm, like he couldn't wait to break their smiles and positivity, before he greeted many of the new racers, though it was with a different attitude, a slightly less sinister one. Most of the group that I arrived with was composed of the veterans. We all knew how this game within the game worked so we waited as long as we could before we began, typically the sooner you arrived, the sooner you were put to work.

That was true that day, a majority of the newcomers arrived ready to go, and they were treated to kicking things off early and had already been at Andy's house for a while breaking up rocks and stones. Many of them were using the butt of their axes. Seeing this technique, I assumed that was what we had to do, which Andy confirmed. I went to work, but not even a few minutes after I started we were interrupted and all veterans were summoned to convene on the front lawn of Andy's house. It was then that we were immediately directed to do some obnoxious number of burpees – the typical "Spartan" 300.

Just then our good friend, Todd, made his now expected late appearance. There's a price for everything with these events – and Todd paid a heavy price! Instead of 300 burpees he was ordered to do 1000 burpees! The rest of us were held responsible for counting for him. That whole *burpee fest* lasted a good five to ten minutes before the race directors became bored with the shenanigans of messing with Todd. Soon after, we were further broken up into Veteran Finishers and Veteran Non-Finishers. Those who had finished – officially and unofficially – were directed to make our way back toward Riverside Farm. I wasn't sure what to expect, but it was back to Riverside having been an *unofficial* finisher the year prior.

Upon our return to Riverside Farm, we discovered what would occupy the next few hours of our life. As it turned out, during some of the camps that Peak Races hosted, the race directors already had participants set some rather large stones into the earth to start building a staircase up the side of the mountain. Sections of the stone staircase were for the weddings hosted onsite and it created an easily-navigable way for the high-end wedding parties to climb to the top of the mountain.

When you think about it, what better way to improve one of your businesses (and the land you live on) then to have a group of Death Racers build you a beautiful staircase up the side of the mountain right there in your backyard. I couldn't help but hand it to the race directors, these guys were brilliant. Not only were they challenging humans at these extreme levels, charging hundreds of dollars for the opportunity (and "privilege") to participate while simultaneously gaining an enormous amount of better-than-free labor.

It still boggles my mind, but I did my best to ignore the capitalistic genius, and focused on something more meaningful to gain from this experience. What we were a part of was quite historic and a person really can't put a price on experience. To this day, these experiences provided me with a better frame of reference and a clear lens through which to view my life and everything that occurs within it. One day when I have grandchildren, that is if I do, I'll be able to tell them, "When I was a young whippersnapper, I helped build a staircase on a mountain in Vermont," and hopefully, I'd be able to show them, too.

The first section at the base of the mountain was mostly complete. However, the staircase was not up to Joe's standards, so we had to "elevate" it. Given the primary purpose of this new staircase (to serve as a pathway to the top for guests of high-end weddings) it was understandable to place a high degree of importance of making it solid as well as picture perfect.

Many of the stones that were previously set in place had moved too much. Other stones were not large enough to fit together in such a way that would cohesively piece the staircase puzzle together with a tight fit. The task of building the staircase quickly evolved into this massively large and heavy puzzle we had to solve. The further we progressed, the more difficult the coordinated assembly of this puzzle became. Afterall, these were extremely heavy puzzle pieces. Each required teamwork, communication, and synergy to get them to their proper place. Every effort, purposeful. And once they were all put together, they would create a magnificent work of art.

One day this stone staircase will be remembered as the

masterpiece conceived by these two outlandish race directors and built by their band of endurance athletes seeking a higher purpose in life.

Much like the Egyptians, but under very polarized conditions, who built the pyramids, we had to use primitive tools to get the job done. Building this staircase into the mountainside was our pyramid. The race organizers supplied us with a collection of iron poles which were handed over to us by a few of the race volunteers. That was the extent to which we were guided on how to get the job done. The rest was up to the racers to figure out together.

Just as we were about to start our new landscaping jobs, a new set of directions were dispersed and they ordered us back to Andy's. We quickly made our way through the single track trail that lead straight from the Riverside Farm to Andy's. Not even halfway there we had to turn around once again.

It was actually extraordinarily convenient. As we arrived back at the stone staircase Joe instructed us to sort ourselves into teams of five. Each side had a captain and Olof, the reigning champion of Death Race, became the central leader of all the teams. I was pretty stoked about our group, we had an excellent team: Amelia Boone, Mark Webb, Bryan Selm, Isaiah Vidal and myself with Mark taking the lead as our captain.

We set to work on the staircase immediately. Within minutes you could tell we weren't exactly sure how to organize and structure a staircase assembly line. Instead of focusing on one task at a time, everyone was trying to do everything from start-to-finish, which just led to a lot of stepping on each others' toes.

The group focused too closely on piecing the puzzle together instead of on how to work together. It was quickly evident that what we were doing wasn't working very well. When Jeff Foster, a deeply knowledgeable veteran, made his way over, he was immediately assigned to take over for Olof in commanding the groups of previous Death Racers in the assembly of the stone staircase.

I later found out, Jeff actually did this sort of thing for a living, so he knew exactly how to delegate what needed to be done and was able to get our asses back in gear. We quickly went from being a bunch of individually-minded Death Racers who were simply moving stones through sloppy mud and randomly hacking away at branches, to forming into a collaborative group that worked together as a cohesive unit.

Now, instead of fumbling about, we were actually building a well thought out stone staircase.

It's a fact, together, this unique and select group of sufferseekers and endurance junkies were making history, one stone step at a time.

CHAPTER 15

MILE HIGH STAIRCASE

"Nothing is impossible; the word itself says 'I'm possible'!"
~ Audrey Hepburn

We spent the entirety of our first night of this Death Race on Joe's mountain and we didn't stop working on the staircase until somewhere around 3:00 o'clock in the wee hours of the morning. From morning until nightfall, we worked tirelessly building those stairs, it was extraordinary to witness the transformation of that mountainside. Throughout the challenge, it was evident that some teams expended more energy and put forth more effort in the creation of this mountain staircase compared with what other groups accomplished.

My personal observation was that, Team 1, the team that I was humbly a part of, was absolutely killing it. Our section of the staircase was among the best. We meticulously cared for each stone we place. Combining a bunch of OCD, type-A athletes, like us, produces a high-quality standard in everything we do. Truth be told, what we had built was something to be quite proud of.

Concerning the weight of each of these stone stairs, the estimates for what we moved were anywhere from 300 to 3000-lbs for each of these boulders. Every step on that mountainside required precise lifting and positioning before sliding them into place. The most impressive of stone steps that we placed had to be the one that one assistant to the race directors, Don Devaney, claimed had comparable weight to that of a Ford F-150. In other words, this single stone step weighed somewhere in the vicinity of 5,000-lbs!

To make this happen, we needed to recruit help from other teams. We couldn't do it alone. This task was monumental and required coordination from everyone involved. From figuring out strategies for: how we would lift the stone, how we needed the boulder to slide into place, how we were going to stop it from going too far, how we would prevent anyone from being injured, a communicative team effort was absolutely essential.

It would be tragic and disastrous should we endanger anyone's life. Being fully-present and focused was the only option. With a bunch of basic and primitive tools on-hand, this collection of America's finest type-A athletic personalities were gathered on a mountainside in rural Vermont to achieve this task. The trick was finding a way for all of these athletes to work together without ego getting in the way.

Nevertheless, to accomplish the task of moving a Ford F-150-sized boulder we needed to lay a few iron pipes in a strategic fashion such that the boulder could be directed and maneuvered right into the proper place. Another pair of iron pipes were placed at the stopping point as a barricade to prevent the boulder from traveling further down the mountain than intended should it gain too much momentum. Once everything was in place, three or more racers pried the boulder up from the ground with even more iron pipes.

Naturally, there were naysayers, a lot of them. But we were confident our strategic approach would work. I quickly took the lead and directed the others with a sense of purpose and direction. Our team had already moved many large boulders, and although they were not quite this large, those boulders were of similar depth. This meant we already established an efficient system to accomplish the challenge at hand. Once the boulder was hoisted onto the parallel iron pipe, it accelerated rapidly, thankfully coming to an abrupt halt the moment it hit soil.

What seemed like a disaster waiting to happen (especially to the naysayers) wound up one of the more successful and fantastic events that took place during the process of constructing this tremendous staircase. The feeling of success felt so damn good, especially because it silenced the doubters. Not only had we succeeded in achieving this, at the same time this single stone connected one of the last sections of the staircase together.

All this time there were only a few things on my mind:

1. Keep going.

2. This is supposed to be the easy part.

3. Don't push myself too hard. Not yet, at least.

4. Remember to monitor nutrition and hydration, staying ahead of the inevitable caloric deficit early on would only benefit me later.

During that whole process, as we busted our asses building those stairs. I had started hearing from some of the racers that we might be offered food from the race staff as a reward for our hard work. Initially, I was struck with concern and distrust of the offering.

"Why would they give us food? Was this a gamble? Were we being tricked? Why would they help us?," these thoughts raced through my head.

Furthermore, I questioned what was the deal with the race staff utilizing a Spartan sponsorship with ZICO to provide coconut water to all of us racers. For as long as this race existed, a large part of the challenge of the race format stemmed from the expectation that racers would be entirely self-supported. These kind offerings of food and water seemed out of place and left me suspicious of their motives.

To me, it seemed like the people pulling strings were helping us and they were acting in a manner that seemed way too helpful for a Death Race. Eventually, it hit me. Until that stone staircase was fully-assembled we wouldn't be going anywhere else. This was something that had to be finished in its entirety.

This realization was profound. The race staff and race directors figured out how to ensure the staircase was completed quickly. Their solution was to provide a bunch of ravenous athletes with sustenance. If the race directors fed us, it would mean we continued to get work done. As we all know, a well-fed worker will continue working effectively. A hungry worker will become slow as they are distracted by their basic needs. The meal was rotisserie chicken, coleslaw, and some bread. It was absolutely delicious. I forgot about my suspicions and gave in and feasted. Then, I immediately went straight back to work. If this was indeed their motivation for feeding all of us racers, it worked quite well. Unlike other Death Races, very few dropped during those first 18-24 hours assembling that staircase.

The completed staircase looked magnificent and is truly a wonder. Should you ever find yourself in Vermont, I urge you to travel to Pittsfield, go to Riverside Farm and navigate down the drive to the trailhead near the Groom's cabin and you'll find the stone stairs. Pittsfield is a friendly town, so if you get lost I'm sure you can ask around and they would happily point you to them. Each year I've returned since, those stairs have only improved with age.

After completing the task, teams were sent one-at-a-time to the top of the mountain to Shrek's Cabin. Atop the mountain we were directed to turn-off our headlamps and to find a place to sit or lay down. I found myself sitting next to my friends from Illinois, Michelle Lomelino and Lee Biga, impatiently waiting for the actual race to begin already.

We lay there under one of the larger moons I've ever seen — it shined through these wispy clouds giving the sky this ominous hue. The moon really set the scene. The view of the nighttime sky at the top of Joe's mountain was incredible. Having been born and raised in Chicago, I really loved to take in all the beauty the night sky had to offer in rural Vermont. All the twinkling stars put things into perspective, I got lost under the night sky out there — and I didn't want to be found. That made me happy — to be lost in a moment.

That evening I took notice that Joe's mountaintop had come a long way since the last time I found myself up there. What was once a bare cabin made of wood and some stones was now reinforced and made more sturdy with the placement of a stonewall exterior. It's fascinating how Joe has managed to provide an environment in which the training activities actually create something that has become useful not only for these races and the racers but for the community and anyone who climbs this mountain. Much like the stone staircase this too was built by athletes seeking a life transformation.

I was soon disrupted from my admiration for everything around me with directions to get up, turn-on our headlamps, and get to work continuing to improve the surrounding landscape. Yet again, we were put to work to cultivate the amenities and surroundings this mountaintop offered. It was time to equip ourselves with our snips, foldable hand saws and/or any other useful tools we brought so we could manicure some bushes and take down the overgrown brush. A few of the racers were instructed to move logs and stones to create a seating area around an impressively hand-built stone fire pit.

Someone instructed me to do some hedging, so I equipped myself with my folding hand saw and began to cut my way through the tall grass, invasive weeds, and whatever else I was told to cut through. Joe continuously reminded us about the wedding that would be taking place later in the day. It was paramount we finished everything on time. The harsh reality, no one ever saw a wedding take place that weekend. It seemed as though they fabricated it to make sure we worked with a focused purpose.

As we completed most of the landscaping, there was this massively large boulder at the top of the mountain that damn near everyone who was in the race were trying to move. With over 90% of the field of racers occupied with this seemingly impossible endeavor, I found myself still focused on clearing my section. I was nearly done. When I looked over at how they were trying to accomplish this task, I could see the ropes were fraying and looked like they might snap any minute. No matter how hard they pushed and pulled, that stone just wasn't moving.

Since I was almost finished, and everyone had started making the request for all hands on deck, I started over to help them. As I began to walk up, I heard a loud *SNAP!*

The rope broke in two just as I approached the group. Since it would take them a while to reset, I quickly went back to cutting down brush. I wanted to remain active so the race directors wouldn't have any reason to penalize me. It's better to do something than nothing. As I hacked away at the brush, Don called me over and instructed me to take my hay and my seed from my required gear list. The orders were to bring it down the mountain to Andy for further instruction. He felt the need to inform me of how long it took him to get from the top of the mountain to the bottom as a reference point, and sent me on my way, adding that I must go as fast as possible.

Quickly, I grabbed my compression sack filled with very wet hay. As a strategy to make my life easier and still achieve the five pounds of hay requirement, I opted to make my hay wet rather than try to carry a large garbage bag filled with hay. Wet compressed hay was far better to carry than dry, looser and less malleable hay. It turned out I was one of the first few sent off on this task, as soon as I had that sack, I took off down the mountainside, full speed.

Determination. Power. Confidence.

I had it all in that moment. I wanted to push myself to compete with everything I had.

No limits.

No torn shoulder.

No excuses.

In that moment I felt more than great. And with that newly-risen sun, I just felt so alive.

This was it; this was my time!

I had been training for this since last year. Even when I was stuck in my parent's house with one arm figuratively glued to my side, I found myself training and preparing for this Death

Race. My mind knew what it had to do. The rest was systematic. My body was programmed to do what my mind told it to. So, just like that, whoosh! I took off, full speed down the mountain. I knew this race was about to begin and I couldn't be more excited.

CHAPTER 16

READY, SET...

"You create opportunities by performing, not complaining."
~ Muriel Siebert

Running down the staircase we just built a few hours earlier was absolutely exhilarating. The sight of all these various-sized boulders all properly placed and dug into the mountainside was a thing of beauty. It was hard to shake the desire to stop and admire the craftsmanship of our class of Death Racers. Collectively, we created a new path that leads from the bottom of the mountain all the way to the top; it was a less than 24-hour transformation of a mountainside — a magnificent feat of human endurance.

As I hastily glided my way down the mountain, I fully embraced the boost I experienced in my energy levels. Simultaneously, I found myself pondering the fact that so many of us had gathered here from all around the country and some even traveled internationally just to be part of this event. Specifically — then and there — at that race. All of us engulfed in a singular task, together in a common purpose to participate in a self-inflicted sufferfest. The whole thing required immense strength, resilience, and perseverance.

I was lost in the realization of how magical that place had

become. It was something remarkable and incredibly unique. And we created it — with our own hands. With sheer willpower and determination we successfully built a mile long staircase.

As I regained my focus on the task at hand, it occured to me that I had already made the trek down the mountain and arrived at the location where Andy directed us to unload our seed and hay. Immediately, I opened my compression sack, removed my grass seed and I hurriedly spread it all about as I laid my damp hay atop the seedlings. Within a minute or so, I was sprinting my way back up the mountain. The weightlessness of travel without the ruck was so incredibly liberating — all that weight literally off my shoulders. My legs propelled my body up the mountain. I moved like the wind — powerful and swift.

As I approached the mountaintop and passed Shrek's Cabin, I could hear Joe instructing Junyoung Pak, "See if you can beat the racers we already sent down and back up."

But, just as Joe presented this challenge I had returned from that task. I announced my arrival to Joe, and he looked to Pak and said, "Too late."

I remember Don being shocked at the blistering speed of my arrival. I noticed quite a difference in my performance from the year prior (back when I was wandering around this mountain clueless as to what I had gotten myself into). Looking back, I realized I was just barely able to get by with that tear in the labrum in my left shoulder.

But that's just it.

Things *were* different this year.

My *power* was back.

I wasn't supposed to be back to 100% and, at the time, I was probably only at about 80% of my strength. However, with all the adrenaline flowing through my veins, it felt like 110%. That was the difference between compensating and competing for an entire year on an injury. This year, it felt like I could crush this race and possibly even find myself in the top three spots if

I kept moving with such ferocity. When I first entered into this year's race, my goal was simple, to finish. I found it funny how quickly that goal evolved as the event progressed.

After this segment, Joe took the first group of us down the mountain where we had quite a bit of bushwhacking to do before our next task. There, we were required to move a few bucket loads worth of gravel to various spots on the mountain to assist in trail repairs. These were the typical "chores" that many racers often complain about, but personally, as a man who came to have a certain love and appreciation for this mountain, I understood what it meant to contribute to its preservation. I was happy to oblige with giving back to the community that afforded us this opportunity to race in this beautiful small town in Vermont.

As we all finished our portion of the trail-grooming chores, we were told to grab a rock, which Joe had to approve. Once approved, he would lead us across some gnarly terrain. Some spots were a bit sketchy and respectably dangerous at times. With all the weight on my back and this large rock clutched by the grip of my hands, I proceeded with extreme caution.

While the terrain was intense, it wasn't enough to stop any one of us. As I recall, I tried to follow the vaguely marked "trails" and at some point, as we navigated, Joe stopped and said four magical words that I had been waiting to hear for well over 24 hours, "The race starts now."

BOOM!

I took off, all systems engaged. I started to duck, dip, dodge, jump, dive — OK, maybe not dive, but I definitely climbed over fallen trees, dodged broken branches, and navigated my way down the rocky terrain that paved my path. All the while, I was consciously trying to pass people without endangering them or myself.

The fire within me raged! With determination as my guide and Amee Farm as my destination, I raced down the trail like a gazelle. Once I found myself on the open, well-groomed trail, I kicked it up a few notches. Still grasping my rock in hand, I flew down the mountain. It was a rush passing everyone, and soon enough, I found myself leading the way. I lead the entire pack to the next challenge.

My frontrunning didn't last too long, however, a racing friend of mine, Isaiah Vidal, saw my speed as I flew past and it lit a fire inside him. The second I passed, I saw him launch himself into a full-out sprint. The two of us floated down the mountain, twisting and turning, jumping over rocks, sweeping through the switchbacks, and doing whatever it took to be the first to reach Amee Farm.

Isaiah took the lead as I started to fall back ever so slightly. I looked back. No one was anywhere in sight. To me, it seemed that we were the only ones pushing ourselves to race. As the clearing approached, I could see Amee Farm in my periphery. I arrived less than a minute behind Isaiah, and I was ecstatic to discover at that point in time that I was sitting pretty in second place.

We were rewarded for being the first two to arrive at the Wood Chopping Challenge. Our reward? We were presented with the most massive stumps I had ever seen! The diameter had to be close to three feet and my objective was to split this massive thing with an ax or a maul. In my opinion, this thing looked like it would be a damn near impossibility to split. As far as I was concerned, these were meant to be handled by machines not mere mortals.

I looked at my stump in defeat and disbelief. Lesson learned, don't be among the first to arrive at a challenge during the Death Race. You'll only be rewarded, no, punished, for showing up early. When you perform at a level that designates your potential to be a top contender, when you're the first to arrive at a challenge, it becomes assumed the last challenge was too easy for you, so you are awarded additional challenges, to ensure that you are properly tested.

As the other racers poured in, I realized that everyone else was greeted with normal-sized stumps, and they only had to split those into six pieces each, which equated to a total of 30 logs to split. Isaiah and I, however, were to split these enormous stumps into 25 pieces of firewood. I was starving so I ate a peanut-butter and jelly sandwich and slammed a Gatorade. Between bites, I worked on chipping away at this monstrous stump I was bestowed with.

Whack.

Whack.

Whack.

With each swing I couldn't help but laugh — it was ridiculous! No matter how hard I tried, I made ZERO progress. Each strike just reaffirmed how seemingly impossible it would be to complete this task. I focused on aiming to strike my Fiskars X27 into the edges of the stump to start splitting it up. However, in actuality, I only mulched these tiny little chips of wood away — I couldn't chop one clean splice. It was pathetic and infuriating. I had no clue what I was supposed to do. I checked on Isaiah, and he was having similar luck — or lack thereof. Nothing would give on these stumps. Relentless with our determination, we continued striking away with our axes, chip by chip.

The other racers trickled in one-by-one and I felt a suffocating sense of claustrophobia as I soon became surrounded by more and more axes being swung all around me. Unlike everyone else, who could easily grab and move their stumps wherever they wanted, I was unable to reposition mine because of the weight.

I even had to ask a few racers to relocate because I frankly could no longer bear the proximity of everything. All of it began to stress me out. I think I even felt just a bit concerned about my life. I didn't know how skilled some of these guys and gals were in the art of chopping wood, and I didn't want to become the victim to a stray piece of wood or worse, an ax courtesy of some butter-fingers. Once I put things in perspective for a few of the racers surrounding and boxing me in they became situationally aware and adjusted their positioning.

Shortly after that, a few of us veterans, maybe 10 or so, were temporarily relieved of splitting logs. Instead we were informed that we had a side quest that involved some ridiculous number of burpees (I think they wanted us to do some 500 or however many). I don't remember why or what the whole deal was, but from what I do recall, during this special handpicked Burpee Fest was that not one of us took it seriously.

We basically mocked the task because we knew the Race Directors would likely become bored and have us do something else. We counted, but our counting was all over the place, it went a little something like...1, 2, 3, 10, 15, 20, 50, 100... it wasn't about how many — it was bout doing them in unison, that's what really mattered. We all went up and we all went down, together, as one.

Now, how many did we do? If I were to guess based on overall fatigue, I would estimate that we easily did anywhere between 100 and 200 burpees, but I can't confirm that number with any degree of certainty. When the burpee torture came to an end, we were allowed to continue to split wood. Finally, I was no longer forced to hack away at that enormous log. After expelling precious energy on an impossibly large log for at least a quarter of an hour, I was finally presented with normal logs to split like everyone else. It was quite a relief.

With the shackles of that enormous log no longer holding me back, I ventured out to the wood pile and collected all the logs I was now required to split. Once the logs were retrieved, I positioned myself on the other side of Route 100 where all the firewood was stored at the top of the parking lot near the lodge. There was a strategy to this, by positioning myself over here, it allowed me to split everything on location so I could go straight to stacking it nearby as soon as I finished splitting all of it. It also saved me the hassle of trying to sling all that wood across the roadway.

There was a beauty in switching from that monstrosity to the normal-sized logs — how thankful it made me. I was grateful to have hope restored for my journey. It was the boost I needed. With that newfound hope, I was able to focus all my pent up fury from the monstrous stump and let it all out on this manageable pile of logs. My friend, Chad Weberg checked in on me. He was nearby walking around and shooting photos, and saw me chopping my wood over here. It was good to see his friendly face. I've always been thankful for the opportunity he provided me allowing me to host Death Race training camps and my own adventure run on his property in Wisconsin.

With the motivation of a friendly face there supporting me, I was thrilled when the logs split like a dream. I sliced through them like a hot knife (or ax) through butter. As soon as I finished busting through all the logs, without skipping a beat, I stacked them and made haste to wrap up this task.

At the time and even now when I reflect back, it was as if I were operating like a fine-tuned machine designed to perform specific tasks — mechanical in my movements and my output I completed this task so quick. If only I had arrived third or fourth, I may not have spent so much time here. Regardless of how long it had been, I took just a little more time adjusting the existing pile, and from what I could tell it seemed like I was still one of the first to finish splitting their logs.

After stacking all the wood and fixing the pile, I tried to see if I could move on, but I was told to continue stacking. I felt it begin to set in. Panic. I started to worry that I would get stuck in the wood-splitting vortex. Unable to advance to the next task. Trapped. I wanted to see if I could get moving. I had done my part for this challenge. What would happen? I could sense my anxiety rising, but I knew it was unwarranted and tried hard to acknowledge that it would soon pass.

Another friend from Corn Fed Spartans, Missy Morris, came over to inform me that others had moved on to the next task and I was livid. She could see it in my face and told me she wanted to make sure I knew that the race directors had started dismissing racers from this task and I should be able to be on my way. I was thankful for the news she presented me but pissed at my current situation. I was mostly mad at myself for not paying closer attention to what was happening all around me. I really wanted to depart with that first group.

For whatever reason, it felt like I somehow got screwed out of being the first to leave even though I was among the first two to arrive. Then, I had to crank out a bunch of burpees when I should have been splitting wood. And yet, I was still one of the first to finish chopping all my logs but here I was lagging behind and not finding myself leading the pack.

How did this just happen?

When this transpired, I was not happy but I had to accept reality.

This was the Death Race.

I knew this type of thing could happen, which was the reason why I had so much concern about moving on to the next challenge.

Trying to set my fury aside, I made my way back across Route 100 and went to the gear tent where Candie Bobick, another friend from the Corn Fed Spartans, stopped me. Apparently, my frantic rush to get my stuff together and catch up with the others gave reason for Candie to become concerned that I wasn't in the right state of mind. That my driving motivation wasn't in the right place.

She asked me when the last time I had something to eat was and I was unable to answer her. My mind raced around trying to think of what I needed to bring with me. In the Death Race, you are never aware of how long it'll be until you will have access to your drop-bin again, so this was my chance to prepare for what could turn into 24 hours in the woods. I had to be ready for any possibility.

My mind continued to race. Did I need shoes? Socks? How much food should I bring? I could barely think and Candie could tell. She stopped me and forced me to drink some chocolate milk. It was so damn delicious, it quickly revitalized my lack of nutrients. She fed me some other goodies including pretzels, one of my favorite salty snacks. I was so deprived and I was so low on sodium, all the salt was giving me the things I needed to continue moving along. It was good. This was good. The food, the help from a friendly face, it was all so good, and I was thankful to have it.

Minutes later with my power restored, I felt more self-aware and I was able to focus on my needs for the road ahead. Thanks to that quick snack, I was back on track. Keeping up with your nutrition is easily one of the most important elements when it comes to successfully navigating your way through a Death Race or any endurance race for that matter. Personally, I'm usually very self-aware of my food intake, but at this moment my priorities were a mess and I had lost track of my calorie consumption. I would have to pay close attention going forward to make sure I didn't bonk.

Before leaving Amee Farm, I finished packing my gear and gave it all one final mental checklist in which I literally imagined checking off a box next to each item I would need. My primary concerns were resupplying my food and water supplies, those were the most crucial. Once I had what I needed, I was on my way to the top of Tweed River Drive where the barbed wire task awaited us all. I was told I could get there any way I wanted. Unfortunately, there were no alternative transport modes accessible or within my sight, so instead of wasting time searching, I simply started running along Route 100 toward Riverside Farm. One foot in front of the other.

My rationale was that if I took the most direct route that a car could take I just might have the possibility of hitching a ride. Afterall, they did say to get there by any means possible, right? That's when I saw fellow Death Race competitor, Anthony, zip past me on a bicycle.

Jealous and astounded at his method of transportation, I yelled out to Anthony, "How the hell did you get a bike?"

I felt defeated and a little envious, but I continued moving along the road.

"This sucks," I thought to myself. There goes my lead. For some reason, I had become obsessed with remaining in a top position and I let my high hopes of staying in that position get the best of me and get me down. It wasn't characteristic of me. I wasn't here to win, ever. That was never my MO. My Mission Objective was to finish — that's it. It's true, I grew up in a very competitive family and I myself was rather competitive, but I knew where I stood in this specific athletic circle, and my MO here was to finish.

I had to remember that was my main objective and I had to acknowledge that my arrival to the wood chopping challenge in second was inflating my ego. Now wasn't the time for a big head. Thankfully, it didn't take long for me to stop caring about where I ranked as I hiked my way up the long road to the top of Tweed River Drive. My mind was refocused on what I had to do. I had to finish this race.

CHAPTER 17

A DANCE WITH BARBED WIRE

The most powerful control we can ever attain, is to be in control of ourselves." - Chris Page

As I made my way up to the top of Tweed River Drive, I was surprised not to see anyone ahead of me and when I looked back, there was no one behind me either. I was all alone. The solitude felt off-putting. The sun beat down hard as I charged up the same path I remembered traversing the year prior when Morgan and I headed toward one of the last challenges. And just like the previous year, I felt the sun's punishing rays increasing my body temperature.

The reality of being alone and still wandering up the road after Anthony passed by on the bike left me feeling a bit edgy. By now, I expected at least one person to catch me since at the time, climbing uphill wasn't exactly my specialty. I continued to climb until I finally reached the last stretch just before the cabin where Chris Davis, an athlete who worked with Joe to kick-start a massive weight loss journey had once stayed, came into sight. I could see a table where Peter Borden sat as he waited for his next victim.

This was the **Year of the Gambler**, and I was about to play my first real hand at this sadistic card game.

When I approached, I saw some racers already playing the game. I took a minute to observe how everything played out. While I watched, I was greeted by some of the Corn Fed Spartans. They came to watch this challenge since it was apparently the one that everyone had been murmuring about since arriving in Pittsfield.

Admittedly, the entirety of this challenge was pretty gnarly, it was designed to physically and mentally break a person. At the top, was a ravine and a drain culvert that regularly dumped water into the ravine. The chasm itself was decorated haphazardly with strands of barbed wire that hung loosely from the roots and were secured with just a few stakes here and there. At a typical obstacle race or Spartan Race, you would rarely see a saggy barbed wire section, here it was intentionally constructed to be less taut. The whole crawl was designed to make you work for it, you had to take this crawl with caution. In all the Sufferfests I participated in, this was the most gnarly barbed wire crawl I had ever seen.

Some sections required choosing between crawling over or under a log — the critical factor being how easily one might navigate their pack across the obstacle. At the top of this crazy barbed-wire crawl was a fold-out card table. Sitting at that table was Peter Borden. Peter was another Death Race mastermind and race director who challenged each racer that descended to the bottom of the crawl and back to play their hand in a high or low playing card battle.

The rules were simple: Aces were high, if your card was of a smaller numerical value than Peter's, you went back for another round of barbed wire navigation. If the card you selected was higher than Peter's card, you move on to the next challenge. You had to complete a total of five laps, playing a total of five cards, alternatively if somehow you were lucky and received a playing card that was of a higher numerical value than Peter's, you no longer had to complete laps under the barbed wire crawl and immediately advanced.

But let's be real here, this was the Death Race. And much like life, it's not designed to be fair. From what I could see, you retrieve your card from the bottom of the crawl and then you played it at the top.

I took my time to get myself "comfortable" with the obstacle. I took off the tactical pants I wore and stripped down to my compression shorts. The heat was a significant factor and I knew this obstacle would leave me soaking wet. We were required to take our rucks with us through the challenge, so I unloaded most of my contents in the safest location I could find behind the little shack. When I closed my pack, I took a gamble — I left a lot of my gear unattended. In addition to unloading my equipment, I took advantage of the moment and refueled with some Gatorade and snacks.

Once I was ready, I notified Peter that I was prepared to gamble. He sent me to the barbed-wire section with my recently-lightened pack. I was to crawl my way down to the bottom of the ravine where I was greeted by volunteers that would present me with my card. Once I received my card, I could scramble my way back up to the top of the ravine to play my card against Peter's.

Let the gamble, begin.

I grabbed my pack and began my dance with the barbed-wire crawl, it was unlike anything I had ever experienced. I was no stranger to bringing a ruck through a crawl as I had simulated this at many of the obstacle course races I participated in prior to this experience. During those simulations I would often go about doing multiple laps at a Spartan Race and would bring a ruck along for at least one of the laps to increase the difficulty. Occasionally, I filled the ruck with beer as my added weight and then I'd share some with other adults on-course.

However, *this* wasn't a Spartan Race and this wasn't a self-created simulation. This was the real deal and what made this barbed-wire crawl so dire was the elemental addition to its overall structure and design. The crawl snaked through a treacherous ravine one that most people wouldn't even consider trying to navigate on its own and here we had to do so with this metal rope of barbs.

I couldn't help but imagine the race directors as they

conceived this obstacle. All standing in a circle under the light of an overhead lamp like you'd see in a some noir film. Under the lamp the devious minds would be at work plotting and scheming up ideas with which to torment participants of the Death Race. From the dark a man approaches the light adorning a brimmed hat tilted over his face, he looks up to the rest of the group and says, "Here, we'll have the racers play a game of high and low, but to play we'll have them climb up and down the slick, gnarly ravine. To play, we make them first crawl down to the bottom of the ravine. Naturally the entire ravine will be riddled with low hanging, barbed wire, you know, just to give it that added touch of 'you may die.' Of course, we make them carry their rucks, for at least the first few laps. The racers will be forced to go down and back, at the bottom is where they will receive their card, at the top, they will play their card. Like Vegas, the dealer will almost always win. It'll be a gamble to remember."

While it's fun to imagine these scenarios that turn the race directors into evil villains plotting their torture plans, the sick reality is that I enjoyed this challenge, a lot. It was fun scrambling and playing this game. I don't know why, but I really liked it. I had no fear.

As I began crawling my way down, I realized just how advantageous my natural flexibility from years participating in sports including gymnastics, competitive cheerleading, and martial arts would be for navigating this obstacle. I have my family to thank for developing my flexibility at an early age. It all started with martial arts at the age of three, that coupled with the fact my father started teaching me gymnastics around the same time in our backyard, meant moving through a three-dimensional plane came easily. Relying on this past experience, my body took what it already knew from the gymnastics floor and the impressive skill set of a nationally ranked competitive collegiate cheerleading team and transferred that experience to climbing and crawling through the backcountry and participating in obstacle and endurance races all around North America. All that experience had strengthened and improved my ability to move my body flexibly through any space, I will always have my parents to thank for that. They made sure to start me off early, they always motivated and inspired me to push myself to new heights, and it paid off!

On the descent, I began to get an idea of how many of us were already here. There were only maybe six or seven of us when I started. I was still in a good spot. As I crawled down the ravine I noticed how this exercise brought out all these natural body movements, many of which I had come to perform with much ease.

I tucked my head down and dipped under the barbs and carefully dodged my way through the barbed-wire with incredible ease. I felt like one of those spies in the movies when they are breaking into a heavily laser-guarded room. I moved under each wire and even picked a few of them up when I needed to, with zero hesitation. My speed to the bottom proved to be noteworthy. At the bottom, I was surprised to discover that the volunteers were two children. The kids gave me the opportunity to select a card, and as I turned it around to view it an unhappy look overcame my face, it was the Two of Hearts.

Knowing the high card won, I was prepared for my punishment before I even began my climb. There was no point wasting time. I hurried back to the top and tried not to catch my ruck or my body on any of the barbs. From that point forward, I was on a mission to regain a leading position in the race. My competitive nature was taking hold, and I let it. I wanted to push myself to the extreme.

When I approached the card table, I sarcastically threw my card down and told Peter, "Beat that" and laughed, almost maniacally.

He laughed and said, "Looks like you have another lap" as he pulled out an Ace from his deck.

If I were a gamblin' man, and I was, I'd guess that 80% of participants had to do all five laps. The thought of having fewer laps was fleeting, but at least there were some signs of relief. After three laps of moving through the crawl with the ruck you were allowed to finish the last two laps without it. That little difference inspired hope.

With the constant awareness and acknowledgment that this was the Death Race provided me with almost 100% certainty that the game was skewed entirely in the House's favor, much like a casino in Vegas except with even worse odds, the best strategy I could surmise was to barrel through the barbed wire crawl with as much speed and efficiency as possible. For this obstacle, my goal was to finish with the shortest amount of time. As soon as I could drop the ruck, I knew I could fly through this ravine. In my mind, I knew that was how I could catch up and pass the competition.

The further I progressed the more my energy levels surged. The energetic feeling I experienced is hard to explain, but simply put I felt empowered like Goku when he went Super Saiyan. What induced this energy surge? I can't quite put my finger on it, maybe it was the young kids cheering me on, maybe it was the support of my fellow Corn Fed Spartans, maybe it was Andy telling me that I could win this thing, or maybe it was merely the fact that I was catching up to the leaders, and at present, I was ahead of the previous winner Olof Dallner and female winner Amelia Boone. Maybe it was the culmination of all those factors. It didn't matter, my energy levels soared, and it felt like nothing could stop me.

This race was ruthless and it was still relatively early-on, but despite knowing that we were probably only half way through this year everything felt (in a sick and twisted way) surprisingly easy to me. Up until now, nothing demanded too much of me and we had to have been at it for a good 30 or so hours. The moment I was free from having to lug that bag up and down was the moment that obstacle was over. I succumbed to the fact that I was probably not going to win a single one of these hands. I just continued to move as swiftly and quickly as possible through the laps. One lap at a time I squirmed my way through the course, I'd have to slide my body over this rather large tree root while still staying low enough to avoid a snag. Using all the different types of animal movements, I aped-walked my way down the rocks, slithered my way over fallen logs like a snake, and bear crawled back up with incredible ease as I completed the last two laps so vivaciously.

By the time I finished, my enthusiasm for the challenge was

uncontainable. I celebrated the end of this challenge with one of my signature "moves" the burpee backflip. It's silly that I attempted it really, but that's exactly what I felt the need to do after spending nearly 30-something hours awake, moving up and down the mountain, chopping wood, moving rocks, running, hiking and navigating this perilous barbed-wire course. I was still confident enough to show-off my favorite variation of the burpee. When I first set myself up to do it, I have to admit that I wasn't sure what would happen when I went to throw the backflip. Fortunately, I had so much power, stamina, and vigor that I performed it flawlessly. I trusted my muscles would activate and I let them take over, my body did the rest.

To tell the truth, I am still a little surprised I landed it (but even then, I didn't show it). I owned it. In the face of the competition, I felt unstoppable.

This race, this was my race.

CHAPTER 18

THE UNEXPECTED

"Learn from the mistakes of others. You can't live long enough to make them all yourself." - Eleanor Roosevelt

After finishing the barbed-wire challenge I had the opportunity to gather my gear before proceeding to the next trial, or so I thought. My next mission required me to head back to the Riverside Farm and wait. Myself and the other four racers who finished were so far ahead that we had to wait for over four hours before we could begin our next objective.

Once everyone had come back together, we would then gather for the instructions regarding our next challenge. In the meantime, the four of us were basically given a free pass to do anything we wanted. The only directions given were to return to Riverside Farm ready to move out by 4:00 PM. With this newly-gained freedom from the race objectives, I made my way to the bottom of Tweed River Drive and to find a spot to rest in the large field just outside the White Barn at Riverside Farm. This was the same area that serves as the main parking lot for the racers and to my luck, Mark had parked his car there.

When I made it back to Riverside Farm, I went straight over to Mark's Land Rover and I quickly found the key he hid just in case one of us finished early. I opened up the hatch and inside I found the perfect tool to keep me busy these next few hours. I purposely packed my travel-size foam roller with the knowledge of just how broken my body would become during this second dance with death.

While I prepared to do some recovery movements, a few of my fellow Corn Fed Spartans returned from the barbed-wire challenge and came over to check on me. They inquired as to whether I needed anything from my bag at the bag drop or if I wanted anything specific to eat since they were about head over to the General Store to grab lunch.

Oh, boy!

The Original General Store is a magnificent treasure trove of local food and goodies. I love that place and I often wish it were closer to home. I was ecstatic to hear this was an option. They asked me if I wanted anything to eat.

"Are you kidding me? Of course, I want something!"

At this point in the race, I had mostly ate a combination of protein and energy bars, trail mix, along with random snack type foods. The thought of a juicy bacon burger from the General Store quickly dazzled around in my head. Barely giving Missy Morris a chance to ask me what I wanted I responded, "Can I have a burger, with *BACON*?!"

Everyone laughed before they hopped back in their SUV and took off.

While I waited, I continued to work on some active recovery by targeting my sore spots with the foam roller. I spent some quality time rolling out every painful part of my body. This would give me a huge advantage so I made sure that no muscle was left unrolled.

Upper back? *Check.*

Hamstrings? *Check.*

Calves? *Check.*

Hip flexors? *Check.*

Lower back? *Double check.*

My basic theory was if I rolled everything out during the downtime that would help to prevent my muscles from locking up. The fascia likes to tighten up after this much activity and I had to keep it mobile. Some of the guys I made it back with laid down and went straight to nap-time. Not me, I couldn't sleep if I tried, I was still rocking-out from the wicked energy surge the barbed-wire crawl and celebratory backflip burpee delivered. Endorphins, you've gotta love 'em.

My attention shifted to being as proactive as time would allow. I knew I had to reserve some of my energy and so I channeled it into my active recovery efforts. The more I thought about it the more I realized that being a leader in this race was less than ideal, especially early-on. Additionally, inactivity could lead to tightening up, so this was an interesting position to be in.

Typically, the larger the lead you take in this race, one of two things happen. The first thing that often happens is the race directors will continue to direct you to perform more and more work. Basically they try to break you down until the rest of the pack catches up. On the other hand, to properly execute some challenges, the directors may find that it is necessary to orchestrate a forced reset on the race and thus will gather everyone back together.

To accomplish this, they will allow racers who get ahead of the rest of the pack to wait and they will actually give you time to rest. While this happens less often, it does happen. You may think, how is that a bad thing? The thought of it isn't that bad, especially since you've been going for over 30 hours at this point. However, the reality is the longer you rest, the more your body is allowed to become stiff and soreness can set in. Your muscles begin to cramp and you feel your shoulders tighten. Your legs start to stiffen up and the thought of lifting them becomes a significant challenge. I could not let this happen. During those hours in the field, I did everything I could to keep moving and stay active. I did everything in my power to keep my body "fresh," whatever "fresh" really meant after 30+ hours of racing.

While waiting in the field, my dear friend, Andi Hardi came over to visit me. She was also about to make a trip back to Amee Farm, where our gear drop was and asked me if I needed anything. I realized this was quite possibly the last chance I'd have to get some fresh socks and shoes for a while, so that is what I requested. Andi also asked if I needed food but I informed her that Missy was already grabbing me a burger — or so I had hoped. It felt like it had been a while since they left. Andi took off to get some of my backup gear, and I went back to stretching and utilizing the foam roller.

In my head, I kept repeating to myself, "I will NOT cramp up."

If you can control the mind, you can control the body.

Just as I was about to go back to my active recovery and yoga, the gang of Corn Fed Spartans returned, and the sight of that burger brought out a pure sense of jubilation. I demolished nearly half of the burger before they had to take off to look for the other members of Corn Fed who were back at the previous challenge still. The gang only stayed around long enough to hand me my burger and wish me luck.

I was thankful for the peace while I devoured that burger. My caloric deficit was quite evident; it is one of the most challenging realities of these multi-day adventures. In endurance racing, caloric intake and retention is everything — it can make or break someone's race and body. The fact is, no matter how much you try to consume, the body will almost always be in a calorie deficit at some point during the race. There comes a point where you cannot eat enough to keep up the amount that is expended.

To put things into perspective, in a typical day a person will generally eat anywhere between 1,200-4,000 calories a day. Average high intensity hour-plus workouts can burn upwards of 1,000 calories. During a race of this magnitude, you are easily burning 10,000 calories per day. Consuming enough calories to sustain your energy can be difficult, you have to play it smart and be cautious how you eat, what you eat and when you eat. For instance, if you eat too much you could produce a stomach cramp, if you eat too little you may find yourself with some sort of muscle cramp due to the lack of nutrients.

My main focus was to keep my caloric intake at an optimal level for maximum performance during the event. With each of these events, and the more time I spent in my endurance career bumping elbows with elite endurance athletes, I learned a lot about what works for others and I also learned to experiment to discover what would work for me. This time around I focused more so on how and when I would fuel myself than I had the year prior. Last year, I learned the most crucial factor to the success of any endurance event is to sustain sufficient energy levels throughout the entirety of the event. Achieve this and you'll smile almost the entire time. In my second year of Death Racing, I realized I still had a lot to learn but during that race I realized the importance of eating more real food, less bars, less gels, and the importance of eating frequently. Basically I just needed to eat as much as I could, whenever I could. The more calories, the better.

The entire concept was quite simple, keep your energy up, and life will go a lot smoother. In an event like this there can be a massive amount of caloric expenditure. To provide you with some perspective, for the 2013 Death Race I weighed in, on average, somewhere between 158-160-lbs the days leading up to the event. No matter how many calories I consumed during the event, I was certain I'd leave the race with less mass than when I began. The way my metabolism works, it's rather difficult to eat enough to maintain my normal weight. Weight loss was inevitable. I just did my best to maintain what I could. The combination of all the water loss on top of the ability to only eat so much during the event, I found I weighed less than 150-lbs after the event concluded.

Once my crew left, I ate another quarter of my burger and put the rest aside for a little later. I didn't know when we might start up again and I didn't want to risk being too full. Throwing up is not pretty, neither is shitting yourself, a lot can go wrong when it comes to race eating, I had to be responsible with this food luxury. The amount of time that elapsed after the Corn Fed Spartans departed and before Andi returned evades me, it's not as important as the fact that eventually she returned and it was with a trove of goodies. She even brought me an entire pizza! I had already stuffed myself with the burger, but not even ten minutes after her arrival I found myself devouring a slice. I was still hungry, the way I looked at it, I figured it was mentally wise to take advantage of hot, fresh food while available. I knew soon enough, I'd be back to dried fruits, nuts, beef jerky, and the backup protein or energy bar I had left in my ruck.

In addition to all the great food, Andi also brought me a new pair of Smartwool socks and my Brooks Cascadia 7's, which were the same shoe I used last year for more than half the race. I was excited to have something to change into since I had been walking around barefoot the moment I arrived in the field. It was a smart idea to take advantage of the time available to air my feet out to keep them dry.

As a part of my ever-evolving endurance racing strategy, I have found that a pair of the toe socks by Injinji underneath either a pair of Smartwool socks or compression socks is great for this climate and event type. For the most part, I only wore my Smartwool later at night and stuck with the compression during the day. The Smartwool provided a solid layer that kept my feet warm, and it also helped wick away moisture. The benefit provided by toe socks is the ability to prevent each toe from rubbing with its neighbor since each toe is individually protected by a layer of nylon and lycra. This simple feature helped prevent blisters and preventing blisters is essential if you want to endure.

Another hour or so passed, and finally, it was time to gather my things and switch my mindset back into race mode. All the other racers arrived at the brown barn toward the back of the property near the start of our newly-built staircase. As I made my way over to the circular drive where all the racers reconvened, I was shocked to see how many people were still in the race. It didn't sit right. Given that I knew the race was about to become increasingly difficult from here on out. With the amount of racers remaining, there was no doubt that Joe and Andy would be obligated to take things up a notch or two. After all, they probably would want to do what they could to increase the drop rate to hit the proclaimed average finisher rate of 15%.

I wanted to be ready for whatever sadistic curveball they might dish out. As I wandered around the gathering of racers I made an effort to catch up with any of my friends that I hadn't seen in a while to see how their race was going. There was this ZICO Coconut Water marketing tent that was distributing coconut water to all the racers. It seemed out of place but I still decided to snag a few for myself. I made a conscious effort to track how much I ingested, this stuff has a high magnesium content and if you drink enough, let us just say you will find yourself digging a hole in the woods. At this time in my life, I really wanted to avoid having to do that so long as I didn't have to.

I was able to reconnect with a bunch of the friends I made the year prior. I met up with some of my Team SISU friends, which included my good friend Daren de Heras who I endured eighteen-miles of hiking with a year prior while our team dragged that damn tractor tire through the woods. That monster of a tire nearly killed us...multiple times!

My fellow Corn Fed Spartans teammates, TJ Nomeland and Andé Wegner, were here as well. Andé informed me that her race was over. It was devastating to hear. After the barbed-wire crawl, her ruck was rendered useless. No amount of "MacGyvering" could fix it. She tried to make adjustments and attempted some quick fixes, but nothing worked. The barbed-wire wrecked her gear and her chances of earning a skull.

I would never have thought to bring a backup ruck, but after seeing what happened here, I made a mental note. The Death Race is the kind of race in which you can never adequately prepare. There are too many outcomes to prepare for and you never know what will be the deciding factor for your race. It can be your gear, it can be your feet, it can be unfair rulings, or trivial mishaps. You can prepare a lot, but there's a limit to everything, especially race prep. At some point you just have to be ready to adapt and come prepared with enough essentials to allow you to be flexible in your strategy.

Shortly after, Andy and Joe hopped up on a rock and began to explain to the racers, the crew members, and all of the family and friends in attendance that the race was about to "officially" start.

You obviously heard groans all around.

This was another one of the mind-boggling mind games implemented by the race directors in order to play with the psyche of the racers. At this point, I sympathized more for the family, friends, and crew. They often were the most taken aback by these confusing proclamations. Most bystanders are unaware of all the intricacies of how the race works and when they hear that the race is only just starting after racers have been at it for 36 hours or so, it can be flabbergasting.

With one whole year under my belt, plus my other visits to the Winter Death Race, I was a veteran and I believed the race directors were using this as a tactic to mess with us. They were trying to see if they could bother anyone enough to make them drop. The race directors had a goal to make this the hardest race, mentally and physically, and sometimes the mind games were the most effective way to achieve their desired result.

I understood this as I had been studying the race closely from every angle over the past few years. Every minute I spent engaged in the Death Race culture gave me a lot of insight as to what the race directors' standard tactics were. In addition to monitoring their iterations of the event, I also learned a lot from my own personal experience with my 24-hour adventure race that I hosted and acted as race director for back in Wisconsin and Illinois to help others train specifically for this event.

As Joe and Andy began to explain our next task. My mind raced, I struggled to focus, as my energy levels continued to spike through the roof. All I wanted to do was blast through the next part of the race. Having spent that past four hours or so doing next to nothing.

I needed to get back out there.

I was ready for my next mission.

I was ready to curb my appetite.

I was starving for more adventure.

CHAPTER 19

BETWEEN A ROCK AND A HARD PLACE: BLOODROOT

"My philosophy is that not only are you responsible for your life but doing the best at this moment puts you in the best place for the next moment." ~ Oprah Winfrey

At last, the race "officially" started, or so the race directors had told us. The next leg of the race would take us up to the top of the notorious Bloodroot Mountain Trail. This was the same trail where we faced one of the most demanding tasks any Death Racer had ever encountered at the previous year's event — dragging a tire for nearly 20 miles through Bloodroot. Nevertheless, we refused to quit then and I refused to quit now.

With my prior knowledge of how ridiculously technical Bloodroot could be I felt a sense of excitement — this would be the place where many would break. The tough part about this trail is once you get going you find yourself going further and further into a remote location, yes more remote than the town of Pittsfield. This leaves no room for compromising, if you start, and want to finish, there is no turning back, there is no cutting corners. The hike combines a long walk along a road that leads to a trailhead for Bloodroot Gap, this includes a large section of the Long Trail, most of which was rated as a Black

Diamond route. Here, there was easily a few thousand feet of elevation gain that we would climb.

To make things more interesting, everyone was instructed to search the surrounding land for a large rock. Our instructions for the sizing of this rock were sparse, but nevertheless we had to meet the unknown criteria the race directors had in mind. All I knew was that they told us it had to be large, so effectively the mass had to be reasonable enough that I could carry it while under a weighted load from my pack and still manageable with my hands, it obviously couldn't be a rock that fit in the palm of my hand, that would never suffice. The rules required we carry the rock in front of us for the entire hike. They did not want us putting the rock in our pack, over our heads, or anywhere else, the only place it could be was right out in front of you. With a few race organizers as our directional guides, it was assumed there would be plenty of people to monitor along the way. Presumably, we'd have to show our rock again at our next destination.

Before I even began looking for my rock, my mind raced through a checklist of all the gear I had on me. I was strategizing how I could use my gear to assist me in completing this objective: bungee cord, rope, 550 paracord - a lightweight nylon kernmantle rope often used as a general multipurpose utility cord by the military as well as civilians, and more often, endurance and adventure racers. I had a lot of ideas to how I would "hack" this challenge. To be a successful Death Racer, one must be a hacker and excel at thinking beyond the walls of the figurative box people usually live within. Paying close attention to instructions combined with clever thinking can give a racer the edge needed to survive.

As I searched for my rock, I saw Joe harassing Junyong Pak. Joe gave him a hard time about the size of his rock. Before anyone was allowed to take off, every rock was inspected by Joe, and a volunteer snapped photos of each racer with their rock. Supposedly, the race organizers would use the photos to make sure we kept the same rock the entire length of the hike. I highly doubted they would actually perform a photo review at the end of the challenge. But then again, this is the Death

Race, and anything is possible. How much a racer was willing to gamble was up to them.

It felt like Joe had it out for me with this challenge. He knew how strong my performance was up until that point, so he had to make sure I didn't get by easily with any challenge. I brought him my first rock and he laughed. The truth was I honestly thought what I had first presented would be more than adequate. It's not that I didn't want a challenge, but I didn't want to carry more than I had to. So far, I was apparently not challenging myself, based on the denial of my rock. Since this first one was not up to par, I was sent back to find another. When I returned, Joe once again urged me to find a more substantial rock because this second one was still "nowhere near" big enough.

I was dumbfounded.

Both rocks were quite large. A least a foot in length and perhaps and inch in depth, it was a solid piece of slate rock, in my opinion they both had what I thought should be considered substantial size and weight. Apparently, my sense of adequate did not align with Joe's expectations. Anxious as to how difficult this task would become had I found a rock too big for me to carry, I reluctantly set off to find another rock. Joe's games were starting to irritate me. My impatience to race continued to grow, and I thought to myself, *"I guess I am just going to have to find a bigger slab and suck it up."* The next section was going to push me. Joe was determined to make sure of that. It made me feel good inside that Joe believed I could haul a larger slab.

When I returned, I presented the largest, flattest, slab of slate I could find, it was a rugged piece with jagged edges, and it was almost the entire width of my body. I knew this was a keeper. Quoting *Full Metal Jacket*, I thought of the mantra, modified of course: *"This is my rock. There are many like it but this one is mine. This one was mine..."*

And most importantly, Joe approved.

After having my photo snapped, I strategically positioned the slab so it wouldn't be easily identifiable in the photo in the event they actually did review these photos at the next checkpoint. I had a distinct feeling people would be swapping out their rocks along the way. I had an even stronger feeling that I would not be keeping this ridiculously large rock for very long.

When I was on my way across Route 100 heading to Bloodroot Mountain Trail, it felt like the race had finally begun just as the sun started to set. Suddenly, while we headed down the road that led to Bloodroot, I felt the air change. It was already getting dark from the sun setting, the clouds dimmed the sky, and I felt a raindrop hit one of my fingers. Then another. Then it came — a full-on downpour.

In our community, there is a running joke that Joe and Andy have a direct line to the weather deities. Too often, the weather comes in and changes the game whether (pardon the pun) it be at a Spartan Race or here at the Death Race. And somehow the weather always seems to play out in the Race Director's favor. Giving them that little extra bit of suck to dish-out without having to do anything other than letting Mother Nature take over.

The weather was just another way to make this task that wee bit more challenging. That was the mindset I had to maintain. This was just another obstacle. I was sure the combination of this unexpected rainstorm and the treacherous hike, which forced us to carry a heavy rock would be THE tipping point for this race. I was sure this would thin the herd.

Not even a half hour after leaving Riverside Farm, I was already growing irritated with my rock. The one I chose was less than ideal, but at the time my only concern was making sure Joe wouldn't delay my departure, which is why I grabbed one of the most gnarly rocks I could find. His plan was working. It was aggravating me. The stone slab I chose had some nasty edges and already pierced through the skin on my hands in a few places.

"There is no way I am carrying this exact same rock for the entirety of this challenge," I thought to myself. *"I'll never make it."*

There it was...that self-doubt.

Uncertainty tries to overcome the mind right at the moment when things start to get too tough and too rough to handle. That's when I said, *"NO! I will not let my thoughts defeat me. I will not let this rock defeat me...not yet at least."* As we made our way down the road, I began to strategize a way to secure the rock to the straps of my ruck. Before busting out my supply of 550 cord, bungee cords, and whatever other rope I brought along for the race, I tried to strategically secure the rock by using the space between my body and the chest strap and waist belt as a holder for the rock. It didn't take long for me to realize that this method would leave my pelvis severely bruised if I kept at it. So, instead I decided to fashion the ropes and bungees to my chest straps and waist belt, and I secured the rock to my person so I could avoid slicing my hands up any more than I already had.

To keep up with the group, I had to give it some serious effort. I didn't want to fall behind those who had taken a bit of a lead, especially since I found myself struggling to get my headlamp situated for the impending darkness that began to engulf the sky. I eventually decided to stop to take the critical moment to fix the straps on my headlamp at the risk of falling behind. It was bouncing all around and it wasn't secured tightly to my head. The short pause would be well worth it in the long run as annoyed as coming to a stop made me.

I paused to gather myself and determine what direction I had to go to continue. I followed a few racers and united with some of the friends I made along the way including Daren De Heras, Pete Coleman, Junyong Pak, among many other Death Race veterans. We all continued through the pouring rain toward Bloodroot.

After some time on the fire roads, we approached a fork in the road where everyone's opinion was divided on which way to go. We spent a fair amount of time trying to figure out what direction was the correct path. I recalled the instructions we were presented with and knew the left-side path was the shorter route. However, no way in hell was the shorter path the right path to take.

Things became a bit more interesting. Half the group followed

Junyong up the path to the left. I decided to hang tight for a bit before making any rash decisions. I wanted to be confident I wasn't going the wrong way. I did not want to risk a penalty for taking the wrong route, missing a challenge, or the worst case scenario, find myself lost with no idea where to go.

After a significant amount of time, a group of us finally headed down the path to the right. It was longer, which probably meant it was the right way. Not too far along we ran into another group of Death Racers who were led by Andy, Norm Koch, and Jack Cary. This turnaround point led to a lot of chaos and confusion. People who were behind us didn't know whether they should keep going or turn around and join this group.

I decided that seeing all the Race Directors together was all I needed to see and let them lead the way. Where the Race Directors go, I'll follow. I thought I knew I had taken the correct path, but here I found the organizers were leading everyone back in the direction from which we had just come. By turning around, I found myself among the leaders of the pack. That's how fast things can change in the Death Race.

Since we had taken the correct path, nowhere to be found, I realized the other guys must have gone the wrong way. I didn't want to get too excited, so I kept this thought to myself and just tried to keep pace focusing on staying with the taskmasters. The further back we traveled the more spread out the group became. I was running with a couple of people and two guys were in front of me and another pair behind.

My bungee cords were flopping around quite a bit and as the rock slowly made its way out. I finally brought myself to a halt and decided it was best to take the time to readjust my rock holster. When I looked back up, I was alone. No one was in sight. I ran ahead a bit more. Still no one. I turned off my headlamp to see if I could spot anyone else's beam of light through the darkness.

There was nothing.

I was alone.

CHAPTER 20

SURVIVING THE DELUSIONS

Rule your mind or it will rule you." - Horace

I felt a little-lost back at the entrance to Bloodroot Mountain Trail. I thought, how did everyone disappear so fast? I tried to keep my cool. There were two people in front of me just a minute ago — they couldn't have gone far, I tried to reassure myself.

I quickly decided to investigate the route Junyong Pak took earlier. Perhaps he was correct, after all. Maybe that was the route to take. Maybe we were being tricked into going the wrong way in the first place. I started to climb up the mountain.

As I still carried my rock, I could feel my heart began to race. I came to a stop and instead of wasting my time searching for my fellow racers with no real sense of which route to take I opted to use the best tool I could think of in this situation — my SOS whistle!

Near the start of Bloodroot surrounded by towering trees I could just barely see the crystal clear, starry sky.

How did this happen? I thought.

When I found my survival kit, I hastily opened it and retrieved my survival whistle. Since so little time had passed from the time I last saw a person (maybe ten to fifteen minutes at most) I was confident someone should be close enough to hear the sound of my whistle. But no matter how many times I made that whistle echo through the woods I heard nothing in return. I turned my headlamp off to search for any bobbing lights in the distance. Nothing. I set my headlamp to the flash setting and started scanning the horizon in hopes someone would either hear the sound of my whistle or at the very least, see the flashing of my headlamp. Still, there was nothing. I couldn't waste any more time.

I ran back down the path a short distance, and I came upon a pink ribbon, which appeared to be placed in a manner that suggested the way was blocked off. I realized that wasn't the case when Norm came up, climbed over the pink ribbon and started to climb up the mountain. It's no wonder why I struggled to find the correct route to take. The path was hidden, it was "blocked" off. The trail didn't shout-out and say, "Hey, take this path." I laughed to myself and thought, *Wow, what another great way to mess with us.*

As it turned out, Norm is an exceptionally fast and efficient hiker. He moves up and down these mountains with ease and at an impressive speed. I don't think he was carrying any weight either, but the reality was with how much time he spent in this kind of terrain, he should be fast. Though he had no extra weight, I tried to keep up with him but I found myself trailing further and further behind with each step I took.

He was cruising and I was losing him. I did my best to keep up at his pace but in no time, the gap grew at a surprisingly exponential rate and I had to call out for him to slow down a bit. He continued moving at his desired speed. Why would he ever put the brakes on for me? *He* was on the dark side.

I felt relieved that he never pulled too far ahead. After ten minutes of climbing, we reached a road where a group of racers were waiting by a pickup truck. As it turned out, this group also went off course and they were directed to wait here for Norm to lead the way. It was evident I didn't have a rock at this point. I feared someone would call me out for it.

Given the circumstances, I made an effort to blend into the darkness while I searched hastily along the road for something suitable to pick up and carry. I did not feel right about being rock-less. Guilt found its way into my mind, but I knew deep down that dropping my rock when I did was the right choice from a safety perspective, and it may have given me a fighting chance to get back on course. As the guilt built up, I just told myself to keep looking. I assured myself I would find something. And I did.

About a quarter mile later I found myself back at it — trying to figure out a way to fashion a harness to the front of my pack for my *new* best friend, rock number **two**. At this point, my pelvis already felt bruised from the poor decision I made earlier to use my waist belt as part of the holster for my first rock. I can't understate the importance of finding a solution that wouldn't add to the collection of cuts and bruises this challenge had already left me with as I began to feel a twinge of pain again. When this challenge began, I thought I was a genius. Now, I realized how naive I was about my quick-and-easy harness.

I thought the combination of bungee cords and compression straps would be the ultimate solution to secure this rock nice and tight to my pack. I painfully learned that was not the case, the faster I moved the more the bungees gave the more the rock would wiggle its way out and the more frustrated I would become. Time and again, I had to stop. It had to be at least four or five times just to adjust the straps and to reattach the rock. The frustration just began to poke at me. It took everything in me not to let that frustration get the best of me.

Eventually, our little group hit a well-marked section, and we were all on our own. I remember taking off on my own for a bit up the mountain simply pushing myself and trying to shake the delirium that had begun to set in. At the time, Bloodroot Mountain was one of the toughest climbs I had ever been on with or without a weighted ruck. A ruck and a rock made matters even more arduous. After 40 hours into this race the moon was glowing brightly above as a light to guide the way.

With each step, I began to question whether or not my eyes were deceiving me. Looking to the left, I saw what appeared to be a racer and as I started to get closer I was sure I could see this racer rocking back and forth.

I wondered, *What was wrong?*

Were they cold? Is it possible the rain from earlier caused this racer to become hypothermic?

Again, I wondered.

As I approached, I closed my eyes and I shook my head. When I reopened them all I saw were some branches swaying in the air.

What the heck was that? I asked myself.

These were some of the darker moments of this race. I found myself questioning what was real and what was just a mirage from the delirium that takes over from staying awake for nearly two days straight relying heavily on the caffeine and b-vitamins taken every ten or so hours. I would convince myself that some things were there even if it made absolutely zero sense and it was hilarious!

Without question I saw a chicken run across the path ahead of me. Perhaps it was an illusion or some figment of my imagination. For all I know, it could have been from the shadows of the branches blowing in the wind. Not knowing what was out there was pretty trippy. Even if the hallucinations only lasted a few seconds.

That is what makes the Death Race such an extraordinary challenge to overcome, not only do you push your body to its absolute max, but you are also testing the strength and endurance of your mind.

Can you stay awake? Can you make the right decisions on little to no rest? Can you push your mind to keep going when your body starts to cry, only wanting to quit?

The Death Race is ultimately a test of the mind, everything else is just there to make it suck even more. But those who endure, those are the ones who know success.

Along the hike, I bumped into Jane Coffey a few times and I expressed to her how I felt a bit off with all the things I was seeing. At the same time, I was running low on water and I recalled the previous year during the Death Race when Andy drank from one of the streams and told us this was his norm. I figured what the hell and filled my hydration unit up in one of the cleanest, clearest streams I could find. While we climbed that mountain we came upon one of the most incredible athletes I have had the pleasure of meeting in my adventures, a fast and relentless female by the name of Amy Palermo Winters. When she came up on us I thought, "wow she is crushing this mountain." I couldn't help but wonder how her prosthetic leg handled some of the muckier terrain that we had to trudge our way through. It was impressive how much grit she had, it was incredibly motivating to witness her determination and willpower to overcome what some would view as a limiting factor.

Seeing her pass me on this climb with a prosthetic leg made me want to snap out of the little funk I was finding myself in. My current objective was to reach the peak of the climb. Lifting my heavy legs while carrying all the weight on my pack and in my arms, I had to keep climbing to the top. It was eye opening to discover how unprepared the flatlands of Chicago and the surrounding suburbs left me, these climbs really took their toll on me. But, I knew once I reached the summit it would be all downhill from there, literally, and I was more than ready to enter the Chittenden Reservoir.

I didn't care if it meant we had to swim. On that descent, I cruised my way down the mountain, successfully navigated through some swampy areas, and I made up a lot of time from how slow I had been on that treacherous ascent. During the climb down, I ran into Mark Webb. I was so happy to see him.

As I remember it, shortly after finding Mark, a group of about four of us all converged at a road. We had to turn around and take another route that was marked just a bit up the mountain we had just come down. I thought I had seen the worst of the sloppy, muddy marshes on that mountain, but they were nothing compared to what came next. Making my way through the muck, I was shocked that my shoes weren't sucked into the abyss. Thankfully, almost as if the perfect counterbalance to the slop, the sun was finally starting to rise and the warmth it brought was very welcome.

It felt like we had been on Bloodroot Mountain forever. I kept seeing houses off in the distance, but apparently, those weren't real either! What the hell was real anymore? I kept thinking that we just had to be close to the reservoir by now, and how I wasn't feeling right anymore. The food I was eating was starting to get to me. It came at me all at once. My head began to hurt, my stomach became uneasy, I could feel my throat swelling up. Why am I getting sick now? Is this a flu kind-of sick? Am I going to be able to finish? What the hell is happening to me? I felt horrendous...

Barrrfff!!

CHAPTER 21

DOWN WITH THE SICKNESS

"At the end of the day, let there be no excuses, no explanations, no regrets." ~ Steve Maraboli

I was in the middle of the forest on the other side of Bloodroot Mountain, sweating, nauseous, and exhausted. I hadn't slept in over 48 hours and I had just spent the last 15-20 minutes vomiting up every last bit of nutrients left in me.

"What's happening to me?," I questioned.

I needed to rehydrate and refuel to make up for everything that just exited my system. I tried hard to focus on my priorities so I could continue.

I had passed my good friend, Mark Webb, earlier and he caught back up right around the time I had my puking episode. He checked to see if I was alright and I stubbornly assured him that I would be fine. I just wanted to gather myself before I continued onward. I encouraged him to keep pressing forward while I lay there just off the side of the trail. Bugs began to bite me and my entire body felt destroyed. My stomach ached inside and out.

"I can't quit," I thought to myself. *"I must finish this race."*

All I wanted was an official Death Race finish. I was proud of my perseverance the year prior but that unofficial moniker wasn't how I wanted my legend to go. I couldn't let this be the end.

Try as I might, I couldn't really eat anything. I forced down some beef jerky and picked myself up to continue on toward my next destination. Secretly, I feared where I assumed this trek would end at the Chittenden Reservoir, an ice cold 750-acre reservoir tucked away in the depths of the Green Mountain National Forest. Should that be the case, there was a certainty that some sort of swim would await.

And to be transparent, I wanted nothing to do with it. It's not that I am incapable of swimming, my father taught me how at a very young age by tossing me in the water and letting me "figure it out". It's one of those things I picked up at a very young age and I was a fish, every summer you couldn't find me anywhere else other than the pool. As I grew older though I developed an irrational fear of the open waters. Seaweed, sharks, stingrays, electric eels, the more stories I heard of people drowning or being attacked, the more significant this fear grew. I tried to get those thoughts out of my mind as I continued my trek. I had to overpower the dark places my mind wanted to go. I had to be able to overcome my fears.

Not even 50 feet after picking myself back up off the ground I found myself keeled over yet again, expelling what little was left inside me before I went into a fit of dry-heaving. The feeling was beyond awful, my abdominal muscles were becoming increasingly sensitive from all the flexing not to mention the 48+ hours of activity that I had already endured.

Regardless of how much pain I found myself battling I continued to talk myself through this dreadful situation. *"You're not quitting. You must finish. This will pass."* I tried to convince myself.

I had to remind myself that after my experience the year prior that had I created a platform for others to practice Death Racing. The Legend of the Death Race Adventure Race captured the essence of the real Death Race in the form of a

24-hour event. I wanted to create an event that bridged the gap between something like Spartan Race's half-marathon distance race, the Spartan Beast, and its sister company's race, the Death Race.

With this 24-hour simulation, I did just that — and produced a viable simulation of the experience. At that event I preached to the Death Race hopefuls, many of whom were here now, that you have to be sharp, aware of your mind's survival instinct, and cognizant that the mind will want you to stop even when you have more to give. For the sake of self preservation, your mind and body will demand you to stop and not push yourself any harder.

You must overcome this feeling. You must tell yourself how capable you are and believe it. You have to believe that you are stronger than you think you are, you have to believe entirely that the power, your power, it comes from within. You have to take control of your internal power, you have to harness it and you have to apply that power to all that you do. I told them something similar and I repeated this mantra to myself over and over. I had to convince myself that I could push through this experience and that I could finish. I kept repeating these positive thoughts to myself hoping to prove my mind was as strong as I believed.

As I moved onward, I tried to focus. But, as I trekked my way through the forest I found myself becoming increasingly delusional. The lack of sleep was having a compounding effect on top of the series of vomiting episodes. All throughout the forested mountainside, I kept envisioning these houses that kept coming in and out of focus.

Were they actually there?

I couldn't even tell, at times I could have sworn I had just seen a house. I'd look to the trail and back and it would be gone. It was mind-bending. Every dozen meters or so I'd find myself spotting another one. I asked others if they saw what I saw, they didn't. I was 100% hallucinating these houses' existence. In my world, they were there. *Sometimes.*

As the Chittenden Reservoir grew closer, I happened to

come across a group of racers who were working on the next challenge. From what I could see, it appeared there would be one more task to complete before we would be rewarded with the opportunity to enjoy a refreshing swim. Along the side of the trail, there was a sizable mound of gravel that had been dumped. From what I could gather, the racers were being instructed to spread the gravel all along the trail.

Once again we were being utilized to make improvements to the surrounding land. Many racers become annoyed with these tasks that seem to just be Joe getting us to do him and his neighbor's labor, but the reality is that we were helping to preserve and repair the very land we raced on. I look at it as though we were giving back to the race and the community that serves and hosts the event. And given the experience this place provided for us, it was cool that we were building a place for others to come enjoy our type of fun.

Before I would begin to gather gravel with the others, I still had to deliver the rock that I had carried all that way to Joe who was waiting for the racers at the reservoir. Along the way, a series of signs gave us confirmation of the next challenge, the first sign mentioned the swim distance that one must complete at an Ironman, which is 2.4 miles. The next sign informed us: *"Lucky for us, this isn't an Ironman. This is the Death Race"*. Naturally, that meant it would be harder. It meant we would have to swim three miles. Immediately, I began to dread the next challenge more than I did beforehand.

As I approached the area, I tried to distract myself and only allow my focus to remain on the current task at hand. Gathering gravel to pave the trail. When I arrived, I realized everyone was taking an opportunity to treat their feet. I noticed some treating hotspots and others swapping socks.

After my experience the year prior, I realized I was quite fortunate as I walked away from the race with some of the better-looking feet. While they were still very disgusting, my hobbit feet actually fared quite well all things considered. It was a high priority to keep my feet dry as much as possible during these endurance events. In an effort to prevent my feet from the dreaded trench foot that I had seen so many experience the year prior, I decided to take this opportunity to dry my shoes and my feet out. The sun was shining brightly, so I took my shoes and my socks off and laid them both out in the sun in hopes that they would dry enough over the next couple of hours.

For the entire trail-grooming challenge, I walked around barefoot. There were a lot of looks and a lot of fellow racers questioning how the hell I was trekking back and forth up the trails on the freshly laid, loose gravel. Quite honestly it felt great. My feet were drying out, I had to take caution with my steps, but in my mind it seemed like the smartest idea ever. It was a simple equation, dry feet equates to a happy Death Racer. It was plain and simple and my feet were on their way to dryness.

Once I completed the gravel task, it was time to face what I had been dreading the most. Three miles of swimming. Three laps, each roundtrip exactly one-mile in length. After each lap, I would have to take a gamble and spin the "Wheel of Death". On it, was a tiny sliver of hope that would allow passage to the next obstacle, the rest of the wheel would return me to the waters for another lap until I had either won freedom or finished three laps, whichever came first. I grabbed my hugely-oversized personal flotation device, a life vest that I borrowed from one of my neighbors back home. Unfortunately, it was the wrong size, and it was just too big for me.

As I began to walk into the water, I tried to remember the fact that I've always been a reasonably good swimmer and tried to convince myself that I would be fine. As my feet entered the water, I was shocked by how cold it was. The Vermont water was still as cold as ice. It was almost July, but up here, the winter lasts until May most years. I walked further into the water until it was up to my calves, there I stopped and froze.

My heartbeat accelerated. Just moments earlier during the gravel challenge I had felt slightly delusional but overall I had been feeling a little better than I had earlier that morning. My breath became heavy and within an instant, a wave of anxiety rushed through my body. Uncertain where this came from I tried to steady my thoughts and attempted to convince myself that I could do this — that I was still capable of finishing this race. I may not have been feeling well, but I knew I could do this, sick or not, I could do this. I kept trying to convince myself I could.

The reality was, I *was* freaking out.

CHAPTER 22

SWIM TO DEATH

"I wonder if fears ever really go away, or if they just lose their power over us." ~ Veronica Roth, Allegiant

I was standing there at the water's edge, second guessing whether or not I could complete the swim challenge when a fellow racer entered the water behind me. It was a Death Race veteran, Keith Glass. He walked up next to me and said, "Come on, Tony you can do this."

I looked at him shivering and told him I was scared that I couldn't make the three-mile swim. We were on the clock, and if we wanted a shot to remain in the race as official racers we only had a couple hours left to complete this challenge. I had never swam more than a few laps at a time in the pool so I had no concept of how long three miles of swimming would take. Even though time was of the essence, it seemed that Keith was in no hurry. He convinced me to follow him into the water and assured me he would stay by my side the entire time. After a little hesitation to take that next step forward, I finally followed Keith into the water.

We swam out into the open waters. The turnaround buoy was a half mile out from the shore. As we swam toward the buoy, Keith continued to assure me that we could do this, "It's just a little further," he would say to me. "Just keep swimming, and we'll be on our way back."

As we swam, the oversized life vest refused to stay securely around my body and it would rise up toward my neck. It's not that it was necessarily choking me, but the discomfort it caused as a result of my head just barely poking out of the vest forced panic to rise inside. On top of that I was freezing cold and began to experience early signs of hypothermia. Ironically, I feared the life vest was going to kill me.

I began to think, *"I'm not gonna make it."*

"I *can't* do this," I told Keith.

I shouted out to the rescue boat that circled the waters, a volunteer that was there in the event of an emergency. Not wanting to give up, I asked the volunteer if there was anything I could do to get a different life vest. He refused any form of help other than taking me out of the race. He informed me that if I got on that boat, that was the end of my race. Frustrated, mostly at myself for coming unprepared, I tried to continue just a bit further, but not even a few dozen strokes further and I simply couldn't contain the sudden fear and uncontrollable shiver that overcame me.

The combination of the bitter cold waters and the illness I experienced earlier in the day plus this whole life vest situation meant I finally lost it. I completely lost my composure and in that moment I lost my will to continue. With no hope left, I asked to be taken back to shore. Keith tried to convince me to stay in the water, to keep going for the full lap. Unfortunately, his motivation and encouragement wasn't enough for me to want to carry on, I was already on the boat. As soon as the boat started toward the shore, tears poured down my cheeks. That was it, my race was over. I was no longer "officially" in the race, and I knew it. I never even had the chance to spin the Wheel of Death.

When we hit the shore, I was a complete emotional mess. No longer was I the tough Death Racer. In place of the warrior spirit was an emotional disaster of a man. I wanted so badly to finish this Death Race in an official capacity. This outcome was destroying me. Joe De Sena stood in this pool shed where he had been performing burpees and push-ups all morning while the rest of us battled the frigid waters. There in that shed, he stood with a collection of Death Race bibs, each representative of every person who did not finish this challenge. These were like his trophies, proof of every athlete he broke and managed to make quit. The swim broke nearly everyone. It shocked me the number of Death Racers, some were among the toughest, that bowed out at this challenge.

It was time for my bib to join the ranks. It was time for me to become one of those racers as well. I started bawling my eyes out in front of this man that I looked up to. Joe looked at me and said, "What are you crying about you know how this works." I looked up and replied, "I wanted to earn my skull, and I wanted to finish officially."

He smiled, "Just go buy a skull on eBay."

"That's not what I want Joe, and you know that!" I barked back at him. "I want to EARN my skull. I've come so far."

Joe looked at me and said, "You know that you can continue unofficially, you've done it before. Hand me your bib and if you want to continue, go for it. But you won't receive a skull."

Somehow I was surprised by this, I couldn't believe it. The option to continue on still existed, but I knew that this year it wouldn't be like last year. Even if I did go on to finish, I would leave with nothing to show that I was able to beat the game that is the Death Race. So I gathered my things, I grabbed my shoes and socks that had been drying in the sun and my clothes that I took off before the swim and I packed my bag. After a short period of self reflection, I tried to collect myself. I walked up to Joe and I told him I would continue despite how physically and emotionally miserable I felt in that moment.

My next stop would be the challenge at Peter Borden's house. I set out on the same trail that we came from and started to head back in that general direction. Not too far after I had begun, I decided to stop and pull out my cell phone to see if I had service. Surprisingly, I had just enough service to call the woman that I was dating at that time. I was a mess. She answered and I went on to tell her what just happened and by the end of the conversation I told her I wanted to quit and that I didn't want to finish unofficially. The Death Race game had me so upset, it made me feel worse by the minute.

Whatever bug or virus I contracted brought out the worst in me. Perhaps, it was the embodiment of doubt? Perhaps, it was a purely physical ailment. Whatever it was, I felt like death. It's kind of ironic, the Death Race, a race whose name had me laughing when I first discovered the website URL was www.youmaydie.com, was actually living up to its name. In that moment I felt like I could just keel over and die, right then and there. My throat began to swell, I felt my glands become sore and inflamed. After I hung up with her, I internally battled myself, within my mind an epic battle raged on. Would I force myself to carry-on, or would I quit. I *couldn't* quit. It just wasn't in me.

About a mile further down the trail, my body decided to give up on me once again. My head became heavier and heavier as it hung lower and lower with each passing step. I could barely stay awake. I was fading fast. Bugs began to nip at my skin, it felt as though I had become their collective target — my flesh the perfect dish for all their appetite.

Every split second I slapped away at my arms and various body parts in an effort to stop the onslaught. I dropped my bag, in it was a can of bug spray. Unfortunately, my generosity the first night got the best of me and it was empty. Trying to find a solution I continued to search my bag for something to protect me, it was reasonably hot out, but within the bag, I found a long sleeve compression shirt as well as an Icy Hot roll-on stick. Assuming the smell would be enough to combat the onslaught of bug bites, I rubbed it all over every piece of exposed skin before switching into the long sleeve compression shirt. I hoped this would do the trick. Minutes later the bugs seemed to stop. No more biting. *Success*, I thought to myself.

Clearly delirious, I hadn't thought of what it would feel like to have a vast majority of my body covered in Icy Hot. Slowly but surely everything began to tingle, it was this strange feeling that existed between feeling frozen in the arctic and burning to death on Death Mountain. At least the brand held up to its name, ICY HOT. This stuff does exactly what its name says it will. It was the strangest feeling, stacking this on top of the pre-existing stages of sickness I had been through, this was quite unwelcome. A stupid mistake on my part. *At least the bugs stopped biting*, I rationalized. And so I pressed on.

Fading in and out of reality, I came to the realization that it was extraordinarily difficult to maintain the course. I kept drifting off into *la-la* land. I was barely able to keep my eyes open, I fell into a daze, and I nearly went off the trail and collapsed. Immediately, I stopped. I took my phone out once again, the battery was almost completely drained. I called my friend Matt Davis to see if he was still in the surrounding area. Desperate for a ride back, I explained to him that I was done. The sickness that was filling my body became too much to bear. This was it; this was the end of the road, I had to pull the plug, no longer because I just wanted to quit but because I was becoming a danger to myself. I could barely walk. Staying awake became more and more of a challenge and my inability to do so was a massive risk! I almost fell asleep a few times mid-hike and it was not safe nor was it smart to continue. Matt told me he would try to find me.

Over an hour passed and there was still no sign of Matt, and of course, my phone died. I felt stranded. While waiting, I dropped my bag and headed back down the trail to see if I could spot any other racers or someone with a cell phone. As luck would have it, I found a pickup truck that I decided to hang around and just as I was about to pass out where I sat, a mountain biker emerged from the trails. He stopped there to check on me.

Though my hopes were for the owner of the truck to eventually show up, the mountain biker's kindness was beyond welcoming. He allowed me to use his cell phone and I was quite thankful he was so generous given how ragged I looked. There I was, freshly dipped in the reservoir but still wearing a dirty pair of pants and top, aimlessly wandering around the mountains of Vermont trying to find help. I no longer wore a Death Race bib to identify myself as a racer and having left my bag up the trail, I looked even more suspicious as a character. I thanked the gentleman immensely for helping me (and for not judging me in my current state). Unfortunately, I couldn't get a hold of anyone and my hope diminished.

Some time passed, and I laid on the trail hoping other racers would begin to show up. And they did just as it started to rain. There was a bunch of us now, and none of us knew the way back. I explained my situation to them, and in the immense downpour, we all tried to take cover. Much of what happened next is quite a blur to me as I lost the ability to stay coherent.

With what transpired I cannot thank those who were there for me enough in these moments of darkness. A massive conversion van arrived and allowed a group of us racers to toss all our gear in and drove us around. The second I sat myself down in the back row I lost consciousness. Drifting in and out it of consciousness, I was in that van for what seemed like hours. The lady who drove the van shuttled the group of Death Racers around making multiple stops. I just recall waking up every so often checking to see if we had made it to the Amee Farm. When we finally arrived, I was the last one to be let out. I explained my situation to a medic by the name of Charles Piso as I gathered my things in the bag drop area. After a quick assessment, he informed me what I already knew — that I was not doing well and should most definitely cease participation in this race. I accepted my fate.

Mark Webb who had dropped at the swim due to severe foot issues was informed that I was done. He gathered our gear and that was it. The race was over. It was my first DNF, DID NOT FINISH, and I did not finish what I started. It didn't feel as bad as I had thought it would. Sure it sucked for a few days after, but many lessons would be drawn from it. More than I ever could have asked for. All these lessons would give me the wisdom I would need if I were ever going to finish this DEATH RACE.

Once we arrived back in Manchester, New Hampshire at Mark's residence I went straight to his guest bedroom and passed out for nearly 24-hours. I couldn't believe how long I slept. Only waking up a couple times to use the restroom. Entering the race, I weighed in at approximately 160-lbs. By the time we arrived back at Mark's place, my weight had dropped a significant amount over the 57 hours I lasted before Charles pulled the cord on my second attempt at the Death Race. When I weighed myself, I weighed in at 147-lbs — a weight I hadn't seen since my sophomore year of High School. It was shocking.

Mark showed a lot of concern for me, saying, "I've never seen you this down, are you going to be okay?" I was sure I would. In order to pass the time I resorted to taking down NyQuil as I tried my best to rest it off until my flight back to Chicago on Tuesday. Mark provided me some of the best hospitality I have ever received. He drove me to a restaurant where we could enjoy some soup, he made sure that I was hydrating and he took a genuine concern for my well-being. I'm beyond thankful to have made this friend and had him there to help me through the symptoms I faced.

When I returned to Chicago, I was still quite the mess. The sickness wasn't getting any better.

On Wednesday, I still felt so sick that I decided to go to my primary care physician first thing in the morning to see what was going on. It didn't take long for my doctor to conclude that I had contracted a bacterial infection.

Could it have been from the water?

Could it have been from all the traveling I was doing?

This is something I will never know for sure, but it's my best guess that it was the water stream I drank from. I didn't take proper precautions and take the time to purify my water, going forward I would always plan to take the extra precautions to prevent such a thing from happening again. The doctor prescribed a heavy dose of penicillin and within a few days, I was back to myself. The Death Race had got me that time, but it didn't stop me from signing up for another go just days after my defeat.

I would return back with all the wisdom gained from the past two years for what I planned to be the final showdown. This wasn't over, I was determined to get my skull, no matter what it took.

CHAPTER 23

THE SPARTAN LIFE

"If you feel like there's something out there that you're supposed to be doing, if you have a passion for it, then stop wishing and just do it."
~ Wanda Sykes

After I recovered from the awful virus that ultimately led to my demise at the 2013 Death Race, I found myself determined to create a life out of this community. This world of endurance racing and pushing beyond my limits became something I wanted to make a part of what I did for a living. I wanted to help others to travel beyond their perceived potential, to help them unlock their own power, their power within.

I was desperate to fully-embrace a life of adventure and I wanted to create adventures for others. There was this compelling need to share the same experiences I had at the Death Race, I wanted to expand the reach and share a similar experience with thousands of others. It became my mission to create a platform that enabled more athletes the opportunity to experience what I did. This was achieved by developing progressive stepping stones to navigate up the mountain. Humans are more likely to travel a path if there are deliberate steps to follow, and we created that footpath with the development of Spartan Endurance. Racers could progressively advance from the shortest distance in the race series with the Spartan Sprint, a 5K distance obstacle race. From there they could work their way all the way to the 60+ Hour Death Race.

Three months after my second Death Race performance, I hosted what became my last 24-Hour Legend of the Death Race Adventure Race. The race was my first big event production project and it was my first real attempt to design my own race. At the time I had the full intent to design it to primarily act as a 24-Hour simulation of the Death Race. I made nothing, but it was a success in every other sense.

Six months after my second Death Race, I found myself sitting in the executive suite at Fenway Park during the 2013 Spartan Race Stadium Sprint. At the time, I had been unemployed for almost an entire year, and without any other job options in sight, I continued my relentless pursuit of pitching my ideas to expand the endurance arm of Spartan Race to Joe De Sena the Founder of Spartan Race. And after a year of relentless pursuit, I finally had his ear.

That day was spent helping Joe with a bunch of random projects that he was at the time conceptualizing, many of which came to light, including the Merchandise shipping containers that you may have seen at Spartan Race events used to sell all the Spartan swag.

Later that night, Joe rehearsed his speech for his TEDxBeaconStreet talk that would take place the following evening. After going through it for me, he asked for my input on how to properly close the talk. For those of you who know Joe or who have read his books, *Spartan Up!*, *Spartan FIT*, or *The Spartan Way*, you know that he loves burpees, and for this talk, he was discussing, "Burpees and the Art of Pool Maintenance." You should look it up on YouTube, it's a great talk.

The premise for this talk was how the burpee is the best exercise, period. In his speech, Joe explains how burpees are the most effective exercise for keeping all of our systems in-check. With the effectiveness of the burpee exercise as his main focus point for this talk, I suggested that Joe challenge the audience. After all, this talk was being held at the Massachusetts

Institute of Technology (MIT), and presumably, many in attendance would be inclined to prove a theory such as this right or wrong.

With that in mind, I suggested to Joe, "Why don't you challenge the audience? Here and on the internet when this video is shared — ask the audience to test your theory. Just have them [the audience] do 30 burpees a day for the next 30 days and ask them to email you back with their results."

He loved it.

The day after Joe presented that challenge to the world, the "30 burpees for 30 days Challenge" took off and spread through social media rapidly. No longer was this challenge just for the small audience that attended the talk or watched it online, but for millions of others who subscribed to Spartan on social media. People all across the world were taking part in the challenge. It seemed like this incredible movement took off overnight. Videos of people doing 30 burpees a day for 30 days popped up all over social media. It wasn't long after this meeting took place that I finally found myself with a job at the fastest growing obstacle race company in the world, Spartan Race.

Within a few months time, I was in charge of building the Spartan Endurance branch and launched the first ever Hurricane Heat 12-Hour, an event that lasts 12 hours and originally took many cues from the Death Race. This event incorporated a combination of team and individual elements into the event format. This 12-Hour event has now been replicated and is hosted in a dozen countries.

It was almost as if it were overnight that I went from hanging out at the gym in Chicago to flying all around the country. I traveled from one race to the next and soon enough my time to train had to be fully integrated into my work. The next Death Race would be approaching in no time and I was on a mission to finish. I learned a lot of lessons but I still wasn't resilient enough, yet.

To become a Death Race finisher, an official finisher, I needed to amplify my existing courage. I needed to continue to improve my power, in running, climbing, swimming, navigating, and preparing for the worst case scenario. And no matter how much I learned from leading increasingly more events, I had to remember I could never stop learning and everything I was currently doing in my work and my training would add to my ever-developing wisdom all so I could overcome everything the next Death Race would put me up against.

For my development of Power, I made a commitment to carry on my person at all times, a 30 pound ruck that held all of my camera equipment, my laptop, and a few hard drives. Everywhere I went, that pack went. During the event weekends, I carried this weighted ruck with me almost everywhere. I wanted to be prepared for the next Death Race, and I wanted the circumstance of added weight to be a non-issue.

My life revolves around training. And while I trained myself, I helped develop and train thousands of endurance athletes. The most important lesson I'd teach them, wasn't how to lift heavy things, or go long distances, no, the most important lesson was, teamwork. In addition to teaching them what they need to know to conquer one of the most challenging races on the planet, we taught them how to work as a team. This entire period of my life forced me to go through some rapid personal growth. I learned a lot about how to get shit done and make it happen, as they say. The reality was, there was a lot to be done, I had to work around the clock, most work days lasting 16 hours. I would be ready for the next dance with Death no matter what. Everything revolved around this sole purpose.

THE LEGEND OF THE DEATH RACE

YEAR 3

WISDOM

"By three methods we may learn wisdom: First, by reflection, which is the noblest; second, by imitation, which is easiest; and third by experience, which is the bitterest."

~Confucius

CHAPTER 24

HERE WE GO AGAIN

"Success is the good fortune that comes from aspiration, desperation, perspiration and inspiration." ~ Evan Esar

The Week of June 23, 2014

—

As the end of June approached in the Spring of 2014, it became apparent that my obsession with this painful kind of pleasure was right around the corner. It was time for another year of battling the Race Directors and myself at the next iteration of the Death Race. This one loomed over my head like a dark cloud that follows the cartoon character around. I felt like I had one over me waiting for the right moment to blast me with lightning.

There tends to be an influx of this constant almost obsessive chatter related to the race that happens daily on social media channels in the weeks leading up to the race. Widespread exposure about the Death Race had reached a new level in 2014. And if you were an endurance racer, a GoRuck-er, or an obstacle racer, you could tell the aura of the Death Race was, "in the air", so to speak. Personally, I couldn't log into Facebook without seeing some 50 or so notifications related to the Death

Race with many from the Facebook group specifically for 2014 participants.

Every once and awhile I received a phone call or an instant message from friends who were entering the race for the first time. Each of them asked for advice. I told everyone the same thing, focus on your nutrition, stay in the middle of the pack, and just keep smiling. Of course, there was more to some conversations than others, but these were the most general yet vastly-important tips I could universally contribute. These were the little things that could go a long way to help you finish, especially if that's the primary goal as a participant.

In the few weeks leading up to the race, I had slowed my training down dramatically after an unsuccessful attempt to run 100 miles at the Peak Ultra 100 Miler that also took place on this same land a month prior. After that unsuccessful attempt, I decided to focus all of my energy on my recovery from what I did to myself at that race. At the Ultra, I managed to complete a solid 70 miles climbing up and down the very same mountains I would soon be running on. After my seventh 10-mile loop I stopped myself from continuing on when it felt like I might cause injury. Ultimately, I stopped for the sake of saving my body for the Death Race. It was more important for me to finish the Death Race than it was to finish the 100-mile run. I sacrificed finishing that race to give myself the opportunity to venture on to complete this one that I had been focused on for the past half of a decade.

During the last lap before I pulled myself from that race, I experienced a sensation that felt like it could lead to a potential injury to the ligaments that connect my shin and ankle. Pain central to this area began to flare up, and it made every step excruciating to take. After the race, I continued to experience pain for almost three weeks and the pain I felt only went away entirely just nine days before I arrived back in Pittsfield, Vermont yet again.

Once again, much like the previous year, I found myself traveling all across the country from one event to the next one week before the race. This year, before the race I joined my partner at the time, Kristine, for a wedding in San Francisco.

Then, the Sunday before the race I flew from San Francisco to Boston to spend some time working at the Spartan Race headquarters. On Wednesday that week, I took a bus up to Manchester, New Hampshire where I continued the tradition of meeting up with my Death Race "bestie", Mark Webb.

Mark graciously welcomed me into his home so many times over the years. I really cherish the tradition we developed. We'd hang out, enjoy a beer, and sip some whiskey before each Death Race. It was a welcome certainty before facing a world of absolute uncertainty. On Thursday morning, we made our way to Vermont to make our final preparations for the race. We spent most of the day packing and checking our gear. Before heading up, we came to realize our combined eight yards of buckskin, one of the mandatory gear list items, would not be delivered as quickly as Amazon promised — a problem we'd have to resolve before our drive up to Vermont.

Strangely enough, as we readied our gear bins and secured our rucks with the essentials to start the race, we both felt less excited about the race than usual. Both Mark and I briefly discussed it and then kind of shrugged off the strange notion. We went over our checklists before we set off for the store to purchase the remaining essentials and a majority of our nutrition for the weekend.

Our first stop, a JoAnn Fabrics store that apparently already had other Death Racers frequenting it. The employees responded with a quick, "No, someone else asked for that yesterday," when I questioned if they had any buckskin. Thankfully, Mark thought of one other place, a locally owned fabric store run by the sweetest elderly lady. When I asked about the buckskin, she didn't have it but was quick to help me figure out an alternative that could pass for buckskin. I happily and thankfully scooped up the two large rolls of tan vinyl, four yards each, and it was off to Target.

There, Mark and I went a little overboard to make sure we had food that wouldn't spoil over the next few days in a storage container, our selection included: trail mix, peanut butter, bread, bananas, beef jerky, fruit snacks, Chex Mix and all kinds of delicious treats that during my normal day-to-day eating I would generally stray away from. When it comes to the Death Race, or any ultra endurance event for that matter, almost any and all food is good food. Unlike the year prior, I wanted to make sure to maximize my caloric intake and eliminate the possibility of coming home looking like I had lost nearly fifteen pounds.

Once we secured all the food, we put the final touches on our gear prep and packing, and loaded the Land Rover up to embark on our journey to Vermont. This year, we were accompanied by our friends James Vreeland and his wife, Amanda. Once the four of us made it into the quaint town of Pittsfield, it was like showing up to one big crazy family reunion. I took one step into the Original General Store and I was bombarded with hugs and smiles from some of my favorite people on this planet.

After a quick bite to eat, it was time to head back to the Team SISU house were I was staying to find myself a place to sleep. It was already late and I needed as much sleep as I could muster. My bed of choice the night before my third dance with Death would be a futon at the top of the staircase in the middle of the hallway that led to the two bedrooms. Honestly, it did not make for the ideal last night's sleep but I was just thankful to have a bed to use so it would suffice.

Of course, it took longer to fall asleep than I anticipated. I wanted to knock out as early as 9 PM, but I did not fall into a deep sleep until it was close to midnight. That night provided me with seven hours of restless sleep. I tossed and turned throughout the evening unable to put aside my thoughts of the forthcoming challenges I was about to face for the next 70 hours.

As expected, as it is before any race I find myself participating in, the next morning came very, very abruptly. My ability to curb my excitement, my anticipation, and the wonder of what challenges I'll face, always leaves me restless the night before a big event. Unfortunately, for me, there was no time to fret over lost sleep, it was time to go. Mark, James and Amanda picked me up from the SISU house and we headed over to the Original General Store to enjoy one of the most delicious and belly-filling breakfasts I have ever had before a big endurance event. That morning, I chose the French toast with bacon and bananas.

Race registration opened from 6 AM to 9 AM. Our goal was to avoid falling into the usual trap of being put to work early ultimately leading to doing "extra" work. To abstain from as much of this extra work as possible we decided to wait until 8:30 AM to enter the registration line.

When we arrived at Riverside Farm, we unloaded our gear, each of our gear bins and set up shop at the Team SISU tent area. This would be our home base, the place where we could find our crew. Whenever we came in for any help we might need throughout the race, we knew exactly where to go to find our people. With all the athletes racing under the Team SISU banner, we had a ton of support, more than I had ever had at any race.

In years past, I didn't always have dedicated support. Usually, I just relied on the support of various groups of people. This year that was different. This year I had Kristine who arrived sometime Friday afternoon and would be focused primarily on me. I was thankful for her dedication and the support of everyone who was there to support Team SISU and the Corn Fed Spartans. It felt good to know there were many in my corner to assist my efforts to conquer the Death Race. These grand endeavors are often the culmination of a lot of teamwork, the finisher may walk away with all the glory, but often there is a band of people that backed them. Their support, whether in the form of high-fives, handing off a burger, or refilling a water container, all of those acts of support and kindness are vital to the potential for success.

After my participation in multiple Death Races over the years coupled with how I saw the race from various points of view provided me with a lot of wisdom to draw from going into this third year. Watching people participate in the Summer, Winter, Team, and Mexico Death Race experiences showed one universal fact — it demonstrated that the participants who came with an outstanding crew often walked away successful. This year, I knew I had that crew.

Note: not all Death Races allowed crew so I only speak to the ones that did allow it of course, but when it was allowed, having a crew, friends, family, support, it went a long way.

Once Mark, James, Amanda and I moved the small fortune in gear over to the drop area we headed over to registration. At last, the excitement I lacked for the event began to feed itself into my soul. I could feel it ignite inside.

"It's about time!" I thought to myself.

It was about time I felt some sort of emotion toward participating in this particular Death Race, for a while it felt as though I was just going through the motions. Now, that the race was almost starting, I finally felt something. I felt excited, nervous, and anxious all at once. It took me almost by surprise. I even mentioned it to Mark, "Oh, there they are, there are the nerves and the excitement...right on time."

While waiting in line for registration, I started seeing more friends. Some included my Spartan Race co-workers who volunteered to help with this race. It's truly impressive how many people are willing to sacrifice their time to help a bunch of extreme endurance athletes set out to experience this remarkable journey.

When I finally made it to my turn to hand over my ID and receive my bib I was struck with the realization that I didn't bring anything else to turn in for registration. The race admins required two belongings to be turned in whether it be your driver's license and a credit card, car keys, or something else of high value. I left my entire wallet at the SISU house, and there was indeed no time for me to go back. I tried to play it off and just told them, "This is all I have."

They wouldn't budge. I had to turn in two items, or I couldn't participate. I looked around to Mark and James for assistance here. At first they didn't have anything they could part with until Mark remembered he had his concealed carry license in his car. He ran back and snatched it up for me. I couldn't be more thankful for him remembering he had that and allowing my use of it for my second "personal" item. Finally, I received my bib number 351 and it was time to head over to the White

Barn where everyone else was gathering for the pre-race briefing.

Everyone had arrived in what became known as the "corral," an area that was gated off for horses near the White Barn at Riverside Farm. We all took a seat with only fifteen minutes left until the official race start supposedly began. I say "supposedly" because remember with the Death Race, you never really know when the race starts or ends.

The year before, it required hundreds of athletes performing over 24 hours of hard work building a stone staircase until completion before Joe and Andy switched the gear into race mode. This year, I had no idea what I was in for. I never really do. Racers just show up and do what is asked of them and I just always try to remember to smile through it all — the good and the bad.

In the horse corral outside the White Barn, Andy and Joe gave us a quick briefing on the race, the importance of safety, and the understanding that medical could pull us if we were not looking coherent enough to move forward. Additionally, we received an explanation that the race would be a traveling race where we would be gone for sixteen hours. The race organizers made a point to clarify that this year would be unlike previous years, this year would be more of an actual start and finish type of race. This year, there would be strict cut-offs. They insisted that the idea of a racer continuing onward after being cut from the race was a thing of the past. Andy and Joe only wanted those who pushed hard enough to continue on. This year it wasn't about merely having the grit to keep going when you missed a time hack. If you missed a time cut-off, you were out of the race. It was plain and simple. The option for earning an unofficial finish, like I had my first year out, no longer existed. I was curious to see how strict they would be if someone were stubborn enough to try to carry-on. At the same time I hoped I wouldn't personally have to find this out.

With only seven or eight minutes left, I took the opportunity to approach Joe and talk to him quickly. After we exchanged a few words about this book, I overheard Andy asking him if they should just kick things off shortly. During the briefing, we were informed that the first task would be to leave our packs and run the staircase we built the year prior, the one we built all the way up to the top of Joe's mountain, and check-in at Shrek's Cabin. It turned out that by positioning myself near Joe and talking with him, I set myself up with an advantageous start location. I stood right next to the closest exit point. Less than 30 seconds later I heard Andy ask Joe if they should start the race, and it was immediately followed by them both saying it together, "GO!"

Thus began the **Year of the Explorer.**

CHAPTER 25

ANOTHER BEGINNING

"I have just three things to teach: simplicity, patience, compassion. These three are your greatest treasures." ~ Lao Tzu

In what was the most race-like start of all my experiences at any Death Race, everyone took off running the instant they heard "Go". We all charged for the staircase. Something about this Death Race, with all the expected variables, felt much different, what remained the same included not knowing when the race would actually start and of course not knowing when it would end. Always the type to keep us on our toes, Andy and Joe had just finished explaining to us that the race would begin in seven minutes. Four minutes later, we were off. Kudos is deserved for their dedication to producing organized chaos.

With my strategic placement, I was the first one out of the gate of the corral. It turned out that positioning myself next to Joe allowed me to catch the last minute intel for the start time change. While I was the first one to the stone stairs, I quickly slowed my pace and reeled myself back in. If there was one thing I learned from my experience the year before was that more often than not it pays to fall somewhere in the middle of the pack versus blasting ahead and taking the lead. Or worse pulling up the rear.

This year, all the wisdom I'd gathered from my previous Death Race experiences would be applied strategically to all my decision making. Over the past three years, I had experienced the Death Race from every angle. As a racer in the summer, as a photographer and assistant to the Race Directors in the Winter and Team Death Races, and as a reporter at the Mexico Death Race.

Certainly, I had the Courage to keep returning year after year to see what I am capable of in these events. I had the strength and the Power I needed physically and mentally to overcome the challenges I would face. Now, I would be able to take all the Wisdom I gathered about the Death Race, all its nuances and quirks about how it operates and pair it with the courage and the power I had developed since this journey started. I would utilize all of these virtues together to finally earn my place as a finisher.

A lot happened during the period of my life when this event became my central focus, in a short period of time I went from a city/suburban boy with minimal experience in the woods to a frequent climber of mountains. I had become acquainted in the techniques required to start fire from all kinds of beginnings and I became well-versed in building small shelters and purifying water. A solid understanding of basic survival became a high importance area of study and I was well on my way to becoming a pro. In addition to everything I was learning along the way, I had a life lesson experience when my torn labrum in my shoulder was repaired with surgery. Months later, I fully-recovered and danced with Death for a second time. In my third year at the Death Race, it had been a year and a half since my surgery and I had all my physical strength back. Over the years I developed more mental toughness than I'd ever possessed before. I still had the courage to keep signing up for this relentless sufferfest that I felt I just had to best, because I knew in my heart, I had what it takes. A lot happened in those three years. It was time to put it all to the test.

I hoped and I prayed that by the end of that race I would earn the fabled official finisher status along with a skull. I greatly desired the privilege of taking home a skull and my bib. Those two symbols for my achievement would remind me for eternity that I had what it takes to finish the Death Race. I wanted that reminder.

As I began my climb up the staircase that we built the year prior, I couldn't help but reminisce. This time last year at the start of the race, myself along with other veterans moved all the rocks that I now stepped on as I ran up the mountain. The stairs we built at the **Year of the Gambler** became a one mile feature up the side of Joe's mountain.

Many racers were already making moves to push to the front. Fellow Spartan Race competitor, David Magida came up next to me saying something along the lines of, "I think I can be the first to the top." I reminded him of our phone conversation a week earlier and assured him (and his ego), that I was certain he could be the first to the top. I reminded him, "Remember Magida, stay in the middle of the pack." He decided to hang back and he thanked me. He immediately changed his plan and decided it was best to stay near me at least for the start of the event.

It's funny but in a short amount of time, running up and down these stone steps had quickly become one of my favorite past times when I visited Pittsfield, Vermont. A month earlier I enjoyed sharing this beautiful landscape with my mother, sister, and Kristine. It was a moment of pride to share the beauty of what we built the year prior. It really is a wonder to imagine that these stairs will be here for the rest of time. It's truly an honor to say I helped build them, not with machines, but with my hands and the hands of my fellow Death Racers.

When I reached the top, I found myself somewhere within the first ten to fifteen racers that arrived. There, we were required to check-in and crank out 100 burpees before we would head back down the stairs to Riverside Farm. The way down required caution as there was still a swarm of racers ascending. As I reached the bottom of the mountain, I began an all-out sprint toward the White Barn. I could see off in the distance that all of our packs and rucks were stacked up into a mound.

As I entered the corral, I was instructed to find my ruck. I could hear Don Devaney in the distance yelling, "If you don't have all your gear you will be disqualified."

As soon as I found my bag I realized the Nalgene bottle I borrowed from Mark Webb was missing and it became clear that they were messing with everyone. Some gear, was purposefully taken away from a few of us. I shrugged it off for the time being as there was nothing I could do about it at that moment and I simply moved on to the next task.

Just as soon as we had returned to the corral, we were instructed to once again hike to the top of Joe's mountain all the way to Shrek's cabin. When we arrived there was no one actually checking people in, but the instructions were to continue on to Tweed River Drive. On the descent toward Tweed, I became a little uncertain of the path we were taking. It wasn't the same path I had taken in previous treks up and down the surrounding areas. I had a feeling that we would make it to our destination regardless.

By this point, I traveled with a group of veteran Death Racers and some newbies, David Mick and David Magida. On the way down we had to do a little bushwhacking which added to my uncertainty. Knowing the general area and direction we were headed, I still had faith we would wind up at the trail that lead to the top of Tweed River Drive soon enough.

Not even five minutes later, I recognized our whereabouts and led everyone across the trail toward the tiny cabin at the top of Tweed. There, a mound of stones and rocks awaited our arrival. My predictions became reality. We would rebuild the sections of the stone staircase that were not up to standard. When we all arrived, there were quite a few Death Racers who had their pick for stones.

I overheard Peter Borden making claims that "If you don't grab a large enough rock they will send you back for another."

I took this to heart knowing Joe and Andy built this entire race off the idea that you can push racers to exceed their perceived limitations when presented with the right challenge. It was because of this, I didn't want to present them with an inadequate rock. I knew that if I didn't find myself a large enough stone I would certainly face some sort of punishment. Seven months earlier, I spent a week helping a friend build the foundation for a cabin on this very same mountain. Joe and Andy had already seen my ability to grind and put in work.

If I presented a stone that was anything less than impressive to them, I would surely find myself facing some sort of punishment and possibly even some form of mockery. In all actuality, I feared that with how close I had become with the masterminds of the Death Race over the past couple years that I might have set myself up for an even more challenging journey. Being close to them just might work against me. As you might imagine, flying under the radar is a key strategy for making it out of this as an official finisher, on the flip side, being well known in this community is like having a target on your back, and there I was painted bright red.

I looked for what I could claim as my rock and moved purposefully. Immediately I was concerned over how quickly so many people had made it over to that spot. It seemed unrealistic for this many people to have caught up already but I soon discovered that most of the racers who started sprinkling in were not sent to Shrek's Cabin and then here, they were able to skirt around and come directly here. An unfair difference in race? Sure, but I shrugged it off knowing full well that everyone will have their own unique Death Race experience. No two racers ever have the exact same race and I had come to accept that reality. It was all part of the culture of the event. Everyone would have a very similar race when you look at it from a 30,000 foot view but if you zoom in you'll see that everyone's experience is muddled with slight differences.

When I found what I thought was a solid looking stone that I could still manage to drag with my rope I got ready to present it to the gatekeepers. I had seen everyone else looking to Borden for confirmation of its adequacy. He laughed at me and said, "Matesi are you kidding me? You should know you need a bigger one than that!"

And for some reason, I was genuinely surprised. I shouldn't have been, but I was. The rock seemed like a pretty decent size, not too big but not too small like some that I saw other people drag. I had a right to be surprised.

Nevertheless, I didn't want to show up with something inadequate to their standard. Instead of searching for a larger one – I already strapped and secured the one I found with my rope – I found some smaller stones to attach that would bring the weight up to par. So I hoped.

My friend, Amie, was right next to me as she worked to secure her rock as well. She gave me a quick hand to adjust and affix the rope to my pack. Once that was established, I began my attempt to drag this pile of rocks I now had behind me. My trekking poles provided the additional leverage required to make myself completely grounded.

With all my effort, I attempted to move...the pile hardly shifted, I could *barely* move it. It became apparent quite quickly that once I was able to get things moving it would bode me well to keep that momentum going. According to science, an object in motion stays in motion and while that may be true in theory, it most certainly is not in practice. Even with the assistance that the slight downhill provided in my favor, the resistance of that pile to move was infuriating.

I looked around at my fellow competitors, and for the most part, everyone experienced the same struggle as me. The boulders we were expected to move were massive. As we all made our way down Tweed River Drive, navigating in and out of racers who were moving slower than others became an obstacle itself. Sometimes I would find this unexplainable energy and I would cruise down the road with ease, but of course, I would only get so far before I'd have to come to a stop. It frustrated not only me but those who followed close behind, we'd both suffer each time our momentum came to a halt.

A little ways down the drive, before we reached a switchback where the gravel road becomes a paved road again, we reached a trailhead that took us away from the paved roads and into the woods. It was here where the real challenge of this task began. The entirety of this trail was riddled with sections of ascent and descent. Some sections were muddy, some dry, all of them sucked. No matter which way I went or how I moved through this challenge, it was a bitch. At the time, I just wished I could pick up my boulder and carry it. But that was just it, the parameters for this task were such that one could judge whether your rock was large enough or not by the inability to lift it off the ground. If you could carry it, "that was not big enough."

Not too much further far down the trail, I met up with one of the finishers from the first Spartan Race Hurricane Heat Twelve Hour. The HH12HR as it is abbreviated is a twelve hour individual and team-based endurance event that I developed for the Spartan Endurance arm of the Spartan Race lifestyle brand. This HH12HR athlete, Brian Edwards finished the very first one I led that took place in Las Vegas. It brought great joy to me to see an athlete I had the chance to help prepare here, competing at the Death Race. The two of us decided to stick together for the challenge. We worked together to pull and push our rocks through this wicked tough section.

After a while I began to experience some issues with the rope as it burned my hands each time it slipped through my already tired grip. I quickly came to the conclusion that I needed to start to work smarter instead of harder. There are times during the Death Race when you have to make the decision to team up with other racers for the sake of making it through the challenge. This was definitely one of those moments. Teamwork was the smarter way to overcome this challenge. I knew this, Brian knew this, it's what I taught at many of my events, work *together*.

I looked over to Brian and suggested, "Let's just start carrying our rocks, we'll move mine and then come back and we'll move yours until we get there."

While they may have made the challenge designed in such a way that an individual shouldn't be able to carry their boulder, nothing in the delegation of the task prevented individuals from working together as one. Brian was hesitant at first, not knowing what the exact rules were and with this being his first time he was concerned with what was considered within the acceptable parameters. I assured him we would be alright and continued to push the subject that this would be a much simpler way to accomplish our shared task. Ultimately, what I've learned in life is that very often it is better to ask for forgiveness rather than ask for permission.

We continued to move our rocks along the path, we would drop them at the furthest point we could safely navigate them to, then we'd go back to grab the other. Personally, I felt like this process put a lot less strain on my body by moving the boulders in this manner. It also saved my hands from diminished grip strength early on in the event. When I took a look at my hands after I removed one of my gloves I discovered that I already had a few blisters forming along with a few minor skin tears on my fingers and my palm. This was not the right way to start a race, I thought to myself. This race would last up to three days, I needed to be more careful.

Admittedly, I think Brian was a bit torn about embracing the new strategy as his boulder didn't give him nearly as much trouble being dragged behind as mine. Nevertheless, we both reached a spot near the stone staircase where Joe installed some new training toys that included a few climbing ropes and the Hercules Hoist. The Hercules Hoist is an obstacle with a rope attached to a large weight or stone that is fed through a pulley 20 to 30-feet above the ground. In this case, the pulleys were secured to a steel cable strung between two large trees. At this junction Brian realized that no matter what we would have to carry the boulders if we wanted to get them where they had to go. You had better believe we wanted to get them to their final destination. We both knew, this was just the beginning.

As we approached that area I could see a bunch of microphones and recording devices set up to capture sound bites and interviews with racers. As it turned out, Marion Abrams, the videographer, and Peak Races Social Media Manager, was putting together the start of the new Spartan Race podcast — now, well known as SpartanUp! The Podcast — which would be hosted on the new Spartan blog that I was developing content for at the time.

By the time we arrived at that location we had picked up

another finisher of the first HH12HR, Christopher Rayne to join our boulder-gang. Chris is an incredible human to be around, always level headed and ready to move forward with purpose. To get the momentum going, I requested his assistance to get both mine and Brian's boulder up to wherever it was on the mountain that we needed to go with them. Just before we could begin the climb, Marion spotted me and she requested a quick interview for the podcast.

Of course, I had to oblige.

CHAPTER 26

RETURN TO THE STONE STAIRS

"Do not go where the path may lead, go instead where there is no path and leave a trail." ~ Ralph Waldo Emerson

In the middle of the Death Race, I was pulled from the action to give a quick interview for the new Spartan podcast that the marketing team for Spartan Race was recording. Marion, the courageous woman behind the Spartan podcast asked me simple questions with complicated answers, "Why was I out there? Why return to the Death Race?"

The answer to those questions was not easy to formulate on the spot. I was out there racing for a multitude of reasons. Firstly, I was out for redemption from the previous year which left me with a burning desire to earn a coveted "official" finish. I wanted to see what new things I would learn about myself during this Death Race.

***

One reason I was there that I wouldn't share at that time was to overcome the many demons that had buried themselves deep inside for years upon years, I wanted to defeat them. By finishing the Death Race, I believed it would help me to quell my demons. For a long time they haunted me, but here I felt like I could bring them out of hiding and crush them once and for all. The memories that haunted me, no more. This was going to be my ultimate battle. Internally, I was tackling an ongoing war that no-one had any clue I was fighting. A demon that lay dormant since my last semester at college. During this Death Race we would end this war. That was my hope.

***

As far as the podcast was concerned, I cannot remember exactly what I said on the recording nor that it was ever used, but I do know that I am thankful the interview took place early on in the race. Who knows want kind of ramble I might have delivered through the microphone had 36, 48 or even 60 hours elapsed in the race.

After we wrapped up the short interview, Chris commanded me to, "Hurry up, Mr. Celebrity."

I jumped back into the mayhem with Chris and Brian, and we continued up the mountainside stone staircase. We lugged and struggled to move what would become another stone step on the mountain. The year before when the stairs were built there were sections where racers took the utmost care to make sure the boulders were set correctly; whereas other parts, not so much the case. There were a few sections where very large and nearly immovable boulders were carefully placed by many working together as one while there were all these smaller stones, easily carried by an individual, that were placed with little effort never fully securing them into the earth.

The key to building a solid stone staircase along a mountain is to make the stairs appear to be one with the earth. The objective was for it to seem as though these stones had been there for thousands of years. Joe wanted these stairs to be the perfect experience for wedding guests looking for scenic wedding photos. At least, that was what I had surmised. This year, we rebuilt the sections that had fallen apart from careless or hurried placement. These sections had a bad foundation to begin when the weather changed and snow came down it all impacted what little foundation existed. Soon after the warming spring temperatures, their overuse caused the stones to become a danger to everyone who used them, especially the locals who used them on a regular basis.

Unlike the year prior, our mountainside craftsmanship would not take the same 24 hours to complete, this time we were not building an entire section, we were merely fixing a few sections. I love the team work aspect of these tasks. Working together as a team to build something that will forever be a part of this mountain, was pretty cool to think about while we worked away. Knowing I could one day return and say, "Along with my comrades, I helped build this." It brings joyous tears to my eyes every time I think about that group of 200 fellow Death Racers and what we built.

It was a lot of work to lug the enormous stones up and down the mountain, but with teamwork and camaraderie, anything was possible, even when it didn't seem that way at the time. All around me, I could see Death Racers working together, making the impossible, possible. The ingenuity of the racers was something to admire. Some racers utilized rope and webbing and so forth to fashion together different dragging systems. Others found sizable tree limbs and created a basket of sorts from their buckskin to carry the boulders. Once Chris, Brian, and I brought our stone up to its new home in the mountain we were sent back to the top of Tweed River Drive to ensure that all the stones had been gathered and used.

On our way back down the trail, we discovered a collection of abandoned stones by those who gave up on moving the oversized monstrosities. As we passed one, we had the unfortunate luck of being in the vicinity of one of the event coordinators, who sometimes was referred to as, "the Task Master", Don Devaney. His role was intimidation. As usual, he began to emote quite loud and boisterous in his angry-sounding, overly animated, Death Race character. What I once found to be intimidating was now rather amusing. My inability to take him serious, often got me into some less than desirable situations. That held true here. Don saw us and immediately directed us to pick up the nearest stone. It was an obnoxiously large one. One that quite frankly, looked a bit phallic.

As soon as Don carried on, we did attempt to move the stone

only to discover why it had been abandoned so quickly. Though in size it shouldn't have been too much for the three of us, it was. Once Don was entirely out of sight we ditched that rock in the woods. It would have made a terrible step, I mean it looked like a penis, literally. Not only that, it was clear to us why that stone was abandoned, and I'm no longer talking about its shape, the density of that stone was so immense it made it difficult to handle. On this terrain the risk of injury just wasn't worth it. Plus, there were still plenty of other abandoned stones along the path that we could move and so we found another and carried on.

We found a couple of racers who were working to move a stone, though with each effort they made they were not moving very far. Instead of grabbing our own stone we decided to jump in with them to lend a much-needed hand. Together, we worked to quickly move the stone that they appeared to be struggling on for some time. It was awkwardly shaped and forced us to carry it in the most particular way. Some edges were round which made it difficult to secure a good grip at times. One foot after the other, we moved along taking breaks every twenty to thirty steps as needed. The pauses we took were short, the primary reason for taking them was mostly to re-adjust our grip and sometimes to give our forearms a bit of relief.

When we arrived back at the staircase, we brought the stone we carried to the nearest spot it was needed. All the while we had dropped our bags in what we had hoped was a safe location. Once the stone was dropped for other racers to secure, we quickly made our way back to the tree where Brian, Chris and I dropped our bags. We exerted a significant amount of energy over the past couple hours, so we made sure to hydrate and fuel ourselves a bit before we moved our bags up the mountainside.

From there, we continued to find others who needed assistance in transferring another substantially large boulder up the mountainside. Our preferred method to move these boulders became based on a rope based system. It [the rope] would be secured to a stone, then six or more handles (also made from rope) were attached to distribute the weight. From there, it was simply a system of pulling as far as we could before repositioning ourselves and doing it all again. As often as possible we would utilize the leverage we could generate by wrapping some of the rope around the nearby trees. It helped speed up the process and we just zig-zagged our way up the mountainside by bouncing from one tree to the next. Physics at work, I loved it.

As we moved the stones up we set them in place one by one and it reminded me of the Hurricane Heats that I had been leading for Spartan Race. A bunch of strangers and friends come together and perform incredible feats. As the final rocks were set in place in one of the lower sections, our group was sent further up the mountain to help. When we arrived at the highest point of the staircase that was being rebuilt, we were told to stop and hang back. It was clear there was no need for more bodies up there, the path was narrow and already smothered by a cluster of Death Racers who worked tirelessly to secure the final stones in place. The volunteer who was there didn't know what to tell us other than to "look busy", so we started moving any spare stones that were not intentionally set out of the way and headed back down a bit.

Shortly after we chucked a few stones off the beaten path and into the brush, we were informed that this task had come to an end and all of us were rounded up by Johnny Waite. He made an announcement that the following names that he would be calling off had done an exceptional job thus far in the race. What that meant is, these individuals earned the opportunity to have a small headstart to embark on the next challenge. There was an opportunity for the racers to nominate a few additional people that may have been missed by the race directors as well. After that those few lucky individuals who were selected earned a three to five minute lead on the rest of us.

Our next mission was to run back down the mountain to Riverside Farm. To my advantage, I knew this mountain very well from all my visits over the course of the past three years. This allowed me to take a few "shortcuts" that easily took minutes off my time getting back down. With a full ruck, I ran as fast as my legs allowed. As I approached Riverside Farm, I saw that there were a few water bottles lined up along with a few other items as well. The volunteers and race directors had snagged some of our things from our rucks while they piled all of our bags one on top of the other. The blue Nalgene water bottle I borrowed from Mark Webb was included in the items they pulled.

As I ran up, they explained that anyone must complete fifty burpees to retrieve their item, unless it was a water bottle in which case it could just be picked up. I ran up without hesitation scooped up "my" water bottle and headed toward the area where we picked up our bibs earlier that morning.

All along the tree line, I noticed there were small log stumps lined up all in a row. There were easily enough for over 200 participants. Some had X's spray painted in black on them, while others had O's and a few even had what appeared to be a capital letter E. The objective was simple enough, grab a log and head over to Bloodroot Mountain Trail.

Bloodroot is one of the constants in the Death Race. You know you'll face this mighty mountainous trail at one point or another during any Death Race. The only question you ever wonder is when it's going to happen. In my first year, it was one of the very first tasks we were subjected to and in my second year it came later in the game. This year it would take place early enough in the day to allow us to ascend in the daylight. How far we would go and what else would lay ahead remained a mystery. With my newly acquired log in my hands, I hustled my way across Route 100 and power hiked my way up the driveway that led to Bloodroot trail.

CHAPTER 27

BLOODROOT WATER GIVER

"So often people are working hard at the wrong thing. Working on the right thing is probably more important than working hard."
~ Caterina Fake

Approximately eight hours into the **Year of the Explorer** all racers left the comfort zone of Riverside Farm to head toward a climb that has broken many a person — the notorious Bloodroot Mountain. Bloodroot came early at this Death Race and it sought to claim as many racers as early on as possible. It made me think that maybe the race directors wanted the length of the Death Race to be something more manageable because with these imposed cut-offs, racers were forced to perform at a higher level if they wanted to earn a skull. I was more uncertain of what awaited us than ever before, but one idea that occurred to me was that a hike on Bloodroot Mountain this early could mean a night swim or submersion at Chittenden Reservoir was in the near future. That would be a surefire way to get people to drop like flies. That swim crushed and destroyed the strongest of racers last year. It was my biggest fear, but no matter what I would face it head-on. If it came.

As I walked down Upper Michigan Road, I started the

unforgiving climb up Bloodroot Mountain and just as soon as we hit the trail, I began to feel a twinge in the arch of my right foot.

"What could that be?" I thought.

I felt disappointed in myself for feeling any type of pain this early-on, so to cope, I did everything I could to ignore it.

"One foot in front of the other," I told myself.

There were a few stretches of flat before the real climb. It was during this quarter mile stretch that the pain began. It was not wholly unexpected since my feet had been mildly sore the week leading up to the Death Race. It was hard to believe but even with all the mental preparedness, I had no clue what to do should something like this happen. For that past year and a half, my shoulder received all my attention. And then that terrible thought crept into the back of my mind, *"I couldn't really be thinking about quitting already could I?"*

This was the internal struggle I faced only nine or so hours into my third attempt at the Death Race. Already there was something in my head telling me this task might not be possible — that maybe I didn't have what it would take to finish the Death Race. As I hobbled on, I thought about the possibility that this issue was the result of needing something nutritionally. I decided to stop near a few friends of mine, Christopher Acord, Christopher Rayne, and Brian Edwards. I ate some trail mix, half of a peanut butter sandwich, and drank some water. It was difficult but I wanted to keep my head in the game so I tried to ignore the pain and focus my attention on sitting there eating some trailside snacks while catching up with some of my fellow endurance athlete friends. The moment of relief was quite brief, it lasted only a short while before we all returned to the hike.

After eating, I resumed my climb. One foot in front of the other, I reminded myself. The whole time I tried not to notice the sharp pain that crawled up my shin and it sent triggers to my brain that told me, *"Tony, stop doing what you are doing at once!"*

I refused.

The wrong side of my inner monologue would not win this battle. I controlled my mind and what I felt. And this, this little pain in my foot, it was nothing. Every step I was reminded that it was something but still, I rejected it. There was just no way I would let anything stop me this early-on. I was too damn stubborn to let anything that, in my mind, seemed this minuscule, to have the audacity to try to stop me. I kept assuring myself that it was minuscule, afterall it was probably all in my head, right?

What makes Bloodroot Mountain such a cringe worthy endeavor is that when it comes down to it, you're looking at a commitment of at least 18 miles roundtrip from Riverside Farm with approximately 3,400 feet of elevation gain. With full rucks, that in and of itself is quite the endeavor, yet alone it was just one of the many challenges we would have to face on this journey. On Bloodroot, there are a few sections where the slope grade is just bloody awful. When it comes to tackling this mountain it's best to just grind it out and stay focused on the objective that currently presents itself to you rather than ruminate about the entirety of the challenge.

I knew it was best to keep my feet as dry as possible for as long as possible in the early stages of this race. Dry feet are happy feet. My focus was to maintain a steady pace so I marched up the endlessly grueling ascent, each foot carefully placed to propel my body up the mountain. My pack felt surprisingly heavy. I was struggling with that added weight of the log, although I never would have admitted it at the time.

I was forced to face the reality that I overpacked while I was in a worried state of mind. When I packed for this hike I had feared how long it might be before we return to basecamp so I went a little overboard. With all the extra weight each step had to be calculated. I needed to expend only as much energy as was necessary to make the climb. I couldn't exert too much though since I had to be ready for whatever would come next. It was a see-saw trying to balance how hard I climbed and wanting to keep myself within reach of the top placement spots at any given moment.

Over the years, I learned that it was best to keep myself from standing out too much. Avoiding the front of the pack and also avoiding the back of the pack was the best way to race, so I developed a strategy to stay somewhere in the middle. The race directors often gave way too much attention to those in first place and it always led to added *FUNishment*, a form of punishment that endurance junkies considered fun.

With that bit of a break and the human feeling of being vulnerable to an unexpected injury, I fell further behind being in that middle-of-the-pack range that I aimed for going into this race. I acknowledged the fact that I needed to pick it up and finish this next challenge with unprecedented haste, or else I risked elimination from the Death Race.

When I neared the point where I had climbed approximately three-quarters of the full ascent, I began to see the leaders on their return descent. I hoped this meant the task was quick and, more importantly, that it meant we weren't headed to Chittenden Reservoir.

A glimmer of hope suggested the end (of this climb) was near and gave me the kick in the ass I needed to keep moving forward. While this was happening, I had forgotten entirely about my foot aching and the pain never returned. Later, after speaking with some professionals about it, I would discover that it was most likely the result of a pinched nerve that worked its way loose because I kept moving forward and didn't quit.

As I continued to climb Bloodroot, I was "secretly" informed by another racer who was returning from the challenge that I would require the freshest of water, and that I could easily find it in a nearby stream. It had to be clean, which meant it had to be from a gently flowing stream. It was important to retrieve it near the top of the ascent to ensure that the water collected remained a nice cold temperature, signifying it's "fresh" level.

I emptied out my Nalgene bottle and filled it in the next flowing stream that I spotted slightly off the trailside. With my more than a half-full bottle of "fresh" and pure mountain stream water, I was prepared for whatever it was that needed to be done at the top of Bloodroot. When I finally made it to the top of the climb I recognized this spot from the past two years. This was the first time I had seen this spot of Bloodroot in the daytime. It was interesting. Now I had seen parts of this mountain at all times of the day and it is infinitely full of life with all kinds of animals and critters rustling about in the bushes, little creeks and waterfalls that flow through the mountainside, and a whole breadth of plants, trees, and foliage that decorate the entire forest canopy. Every time I came here, it seemed like there was always something new to discover: a hidden creek, a fallen tree, the colors and the ever-changing landscape. It's something special to behold. When I'm on that mountain, as brutal as the climb is, I treasure every moment.

To my surprise, there were a lot of racers at the top already. I began questioning myself on how I'd fallen so far behind. It seemed impossible that this many people arrived before me. It was a moment where I remembered every racer's Death Race is uniquely theirs. Instead of letting my subjective position in the race bother me, I proceeded to move forward with determination to finish whatever it was that our Task Master, Don Devaney, would have in store for me.

I could see everyone around me making containers out of their logs to hold what appeared to be a cup worth of water. Some were carving into the wood to create a hole while others built a structure with twigs and duct tape to make a bowl shape that could hold the water. I wondered if that was part of the reason you need to get instructions from Don. Perhaps he was telling people which way they were required to make their container. I waited in line patiently to see Don for my instructions. With the sun beginning to set the bugs came out quickly and they were relentless. I was getting attacked on my face and my arms. I pulled my Team SISU buff over my face. I blocked everything possible and at the same time I was jokingly hiding my identity from Don.

After a few minutes passed Don called all the newest arrivals up to the front to hear their instructions. As I walked up, he looked directly at me and told me to go to the back of the line. He waited for me to leave before telling that group the instructions. I ran back to the end of the line and began the process again. I had a feeling Don was going to be out to get me every chance he could, but I was ready for whatever he had to dish. As I made my way back up to the front of the line for my second attempt to receive the instructions, I had a feeling in my gut I might get stuck here longer than I'd like. This task would become increasingly more difficult if the daylight vanished.

As I walked up to Don, once again I was promptly greeted with dismissal from the group and sentenced to a return to the back of the line. I knew Don was trying to get under my skin, so I refused to let him. It irked me to keep playing this game and wasting time, but this was no big deal in the grand scheme of things. I told myself to remain calm and not show him how I felt.

The next time I returned to him, he told me to reveal myself if I wish to hear his instructions. "Ah ha." He was "offended" by my face mask. So once again I returned to the back of the line. Only this time I would return without the Buff hiding my face. At long last, Don looked to me and presented me with my task. I must bring him the freshest water in a cup sized vessel made from my log. Apparently, he wasn't a fan of my mask, so letting a few bugs bite my face was all it took to proceed.

I quickly headed back to where I had set my bag down next to Brian and I sat myself down on the ground determined to get this challenge over with quickly. At first, I focused on attempting to carve a cup into the log, by utilizing a combination of my KaBar knife, the hatchet Rob Barger lent me and a utility knife. I quickly realized how silly it was to be working this hard to create a cup when plenty of people were succeeding with making the pathetic looking twigs and duct tape walls that increased the "height" of the logs "walls". If it worked for them then certainly I should have a shot at it working for me.

The sun was really starting to drop fast now and I really wanted to be on my way back. I asked for help from someone nearby to hold the sticks in place while I wrapped my decorative duct tape (that's right, this was not just any ol' duct tape, it was white with little black mustaches all over it) around the twigs that I wanted to attach to my log. I poured a small amount of water into a plastic Ziploc bag and set it inside the crafty log holder. I presented my creation to Don, he drank the cold water from the stream, and I was free to go. I packed my log into my ruck and repacked all my tools. I wished Brian good luck and assured him that we'd meet up again. I turned on my headlamp and took off down the mountain.

CHAPTER 28

POCAHONTAS AND PORCUPINE QUILLS

"The superior man is modest in his speech, but exceeds in his actions."
~ Confucius

With the remains of my creation packed tightly away, I took off down the mountain trail. The radiance of the sun faded and was replaced by the starry skies that cloak central Vermont in late June, the first night of the Death Race had finally begun.

Darkness engulfed the sky. These moments are a true test of willpower and determination. Naturally, when the sun fades away the body, and more importantly, the mind, desire to sleep, rest, and comfort. These long, dark hours are a test of perseverance. Enduring the darkness and doubt brings its own reward — like the rising sun's power to bring a spiritual resurgence (and provide the kick in the ass necessary to carry on).

I was unaware of what lay ahead for our first evening alone in the mountains. I just knew I had to maintain my focus on my ultimate objective, finishing. At that time, I knew Kristine had finally arrived. At this point in our relationship, it would be tough when I finally saw her to not to want to stop the race and spend all my time in the majestic wilderness alone with her. Internally my emotions within were all over the place, and as much as I wanted to suspend time and stop racing to be with her, I was equally giddy with excitement at the prospect of having her see what I was made of. Of course, I had my own reasons for wanting to finish the race, but I also wanted to prove to her that I had the gusto to finish the Death Race.

My trek down Bloodroot Mountain was far better than my ascent. I no longer felt any foot pain. In fact, I almost completely forgot about the whole episode. I was determined to return to the White Barn at Riverside Farm to catch my lady. Fire within me began to rage. I barreled my way down the treacherous trails. With my Black Diamond Icon headlamp lighting the treelines up with the power of 200 lumens, it was like I had my own personal sun. With this brilliant light I was able to leap over every obstacle that lay in my path. I could see everything. Utilizing my trekking poles, I navigated the dark path and propelled myself over any water obstacles I encountered.

The further down the mountain I made it, the more I felt the weight of my pack agitating my shoulders. It didn't take long for the aches to interrupt my every thought. In an effort to quell the discomfort, I messed around with my straps. I loosened and tightened them trying to find the right spot. At times I would unclip the chest strap to allow my shoulder straps to fall off which put a majority of the weight into my waist belt.

Even through all the discomfort, I was resolute to keep my pace. I didn't want to stop. By this point, I had made it down the more treacherous parts of the trail but no matter how much I shifted and adjusted the pack, the nearly 70-lbs of weight was just too much to bare. I eventually caved and dropped my ruck on the ground. I had to rest, if only for a minute. Fellow Death Racers passed by and I felt a sense of defeat. I was unhappy with my inability to tolerate the weight. It was my own fault. Even with all my knowledge from previous races, I made a mistake and over-packed.

The truth of the matter was that I feared Bloodroot. In my experience, going to Bloodroot typically meant a trek to Chittenden Reservoir. A journey to those parts meant long-distance swims in frigid waters. Swimming, I can do. In freezing, open waters? That's when I get a little shaky. Thankfully, it seemed we avoided that waterhole of misery, at least for now.

While I continued to make the long hike back, I relished in the fact that gravity was doing a portion of the work.

"Just a little further and I'll be back," I told myself.

It seemed like it was this never-ending hike. As I made my way off the trail and back onto the road that leads to Upper Michigan Road, I headed back towards the path that led past a Spartan colleagues home. I paused to soak in my surroundings.

I was still in the beginning stages of another Death Race adventure, and yet, if only for a moment, it was a chance to acknowledge the vastness of the universe. I gazed up at the blackening abyss over the clear Vermont sky. It was speckled with these beautiful blinking beams of light that traveled lightyears just to reach my eyes at that very moment. The experience was transcendent. Staring out at the expanse of the universe gave me this assurance and reminder that as difficult as anything I might face ahead might be, there are far more significant challenges being faced everywhere else in the world. This was a First World Problem, a voluntary participation in manufactured adversity.

For a moment, it was as though my consciousness expanded and I soaked in all that I am, all that we are, and all that we could be. I returned my mind back to planet Earth after sitting for a brief moment on a roadside guardrail, lost in a stare at the stars above. I redirected my sense of enlightenment back to the task at-hand, I was on a mission to get through this Death Race as a finisher. This was it, everything I had done over the past few years had led to this defining race. You'd be mistaken if you thought it was only about racing against others. The truth is the Death Race is you against you. I was there racing against myself. The Death Race asks of you, can you overcome whatever demons might reveal themselves?

I *believed* I not only *could*, but **would**.

I had to — it was my only option.

I had spent hundreds of hours working to vanquish my demons. Here, in the middle of the Death Race, I found myself relentlessly attempting to overcome one fabricated adversity after another. Personally, it was all in an attempt to destroy some of my own demons. That was the real reason why I kept coming back for more. It was this constant battle with "death" that merely served as a metaphor for the internal battle I fought with the thought of death on a daily basis.

The constant fight against all the shit that filled my head. I was just chipping away at the parasite that insisted on tearing me apart. I knew that if I could finish all of this, if I could overcome all this *purposeful* suffering, it meant I could overcome all the pain that had me constantly at odds against thoughts of a premature death. The Death Race was putting me in a position that allowed me to understand how powerful my mind and body truly were. It was through this experience that I was opening my mind to the reality of my own strength. The fact was, I was stronger than my most negative thoughts.

It turned out that all this time I had been trying to displace these memories, the thoughts of suicide, the feelings of inadequacy, the night terrors, the flashes of the assault, I was burying them in a shallow grave instead of facing them head on. Though you may never forget the very things that haunt you, you can find peace with them. What it takes is overcoming one seemingly impossible objective to realize you have everything needed within to overcome obstacles that are seemingly impossible to overcome. Just like life, it's all about perspective and with the Death Race I had finally gained that perspective. In time, I would realize the Death Race equipped me with the knowledge and wisdom I would need to overcome my darkest demons.

Not too long after my short meditation, I gained a bit of pep in my step. Finally, I could see the lights of Riverside Farm in my sights. All I had to do was safely cross Route 100 and run up the driveway. As I approached the farm, excitement filled me. Having already raced for well over 12 hours; I finally got to see the beaming smile of Kristine. As I ran up, she greeted me already prepared to help me as my crew in any way possible.

I was informed I had to speak to the woman by the teepee tent in the back corner of the corral where a significant amount of Death Racers were already hard at work on the next task.

The next task required me to take the log that I had carried back from Bloodroot and I had to make a hole in the center of it. The woman resembled a traditional Native American woman in the garb that adorned her. I was required to show her that the mandatory porcupine quill could slide down through the hole in the middle. It sounded like a simple enough task. Before I was allowed to do that task, however, I had to change my clothes. It was time to take the four yards of buckskin, or in my case vinyl that looked the color of buckskin but felt like "pleather," and create a top and bottom that mimicked her look. Specifically, I would need to use 108 stitches to create the outfit. Those were the instructions I was given. One hundred eight stitches. No more, no less.

Immediately, I ran back to where I dropped my pack by Kristine and suddenly my attitude changed. The temperature dropped fast, and I was not in the mood to sew a stupid outfit that I would have to wear for what at worst could be the rest of the damn race. All I could think was, how miserable it was going to be to wear that plasticy material. The drowning negativity overwhelmed me. It engulfed my soul so quickly, I actually thought about quitting.

"Why the fuck do I have to do this bullshit? I could just go back to the hotel and enjoy Vermont for once, why am I putting up with stupid shit like this."

It's incredible how fast the negativity can exasperate into an uncontrollable fury. Kristine tried to encourage me that this was only the first night. I had to snap out of it. This is what the Race Directors wanted. They wanted to get a rise out of us and they tried to break those of us who lacked patience. It's not always the physical tasks that will get you in the Death Race, it's the ones that require mental solitude, perseverance, patience.

More often than anything else it's these challenges that force a Death Racer to quit.

This would be my most significant challenge — overcoming the mind-numbing task of sewing, which I'm pretty awful at, my own hunter/gatherer style outfit. I decided to slice the fabric in half to start, I figured I could use one part to make a skirt of sorts or a kilt, if you will. For the top, I would fold it in half, and by using my Ka-Bar I turned it into a tunic, I shaped a hole that may have been a little bit larger than necessary for my head to go through.

I sealed up the sides a bit to fulfill the requirements of having stitches and made sure to count each stitch one by one, an impressive test of focus. Stitch, count, stitch, count. It was a repetitive task that had to be done precisely for my fear of a penalty. By the time I had my tunic and skirt all stitched up I had regained my composure and desire to race. I decided if I was going to deal with wearing this I might as well have a little fun with it, so I took my knife and sliced some stylish cuts into the skirt to give it a more "Gladiator" style look (at least that's what I pictured it looking like). When I finished, it looked far from the garb of a gladiator, but it certainly gave me and everyone else a laugh, that included the woman in Native American dress. I figured it was good to be in her graces, I had no idea how involved she would be in the remainder of the race.

Once my attire was complete, I had to get to work on my log. While the task seemed like it would be easy at first, I quickly realized the difficulty of the task. Strategizing with my crew, Patrick Mies, a fellow Death Racer with whom I had raced with the previous summer, suggested first to begin splitting the wood with my hatchet without breaking it in half. Then he encouraged that I could shove a screwdriver or something similar down the middle. While I loved his suggestion, there was one problem, I didn't have a screwdriver or anything like that. Not even two minutes later, I found one on the ground by my side. You know, it's strange how items will somehow just appear out of thin air right when you need them most at a Death Race.

I worked hastily away at splintering my log. I jammed the screwdriver into my already half split log and started pounding it down with the back of the hatchet I borrowed from another fellow Death Racer, Rob Barger. Once it was through I went to pull it back out of the log. It was stuck! Shit?! What do I do? I could feel my heart rate accelerate.

"I'm screwed." I thought. I threw my log on the ground, then I pulled at it, then I twisted it, I did whatever I could to try to wiggle it free. After I tirelessly worked to de-wedge it for a solid 10 minutes I finally succeeded.

Now, I just had to make sure I could get the porcupine quill through. It was important to me to test that I could do it before I went and showed them. My first attempt I lost my quill in the wood shavings and debris. I had to make it smoother. Enter round two with the screwdriver, thankfully this time it went a little smoother than the first and I made a smoother channel for the porcupine quill to travel through. I lost another quill, I only had two more left. Thankfully, I finally succeeded. It's a good thing I tested it before I went over to show it off. Excited that I finally succeeded, I ran over to the teepee tent next to the fire that was burning in front of it and I presented my project. Success came only after my log almost fell apart, just a sliver of bark held it all together. Ecstatic to be done with that series of tedious tasks, I ran over to Kristine and Patrick to gather my things to prepare for what lay ahead.

CHAPTER 29

CHARRED AXES AND A BUCKET FULL OF LIES

"Never limit yourself because of others' limited imagination; never limit others because of your own limited imagination."
~ Mae C. Jemison

Wearing my freshly-made "buckskin" garb, I gathered my gear so I could begin the next series of events. After I meticulously crafted that buckskin garb with precisely 108 stitches and completed the tedious task of sliding a porcupine quill through the center of my log, I emptied my pack of those items. My load was noticeably lighter. Since I no longer needed the log I was allowed to toss it in the fire near the teepee. This was a huge relief from all the weight I struggled with during the hike up and down Bloodroot Mountain. The next task would involve more hiking. We were to follow a sparsely-marked trail along a snowmobile route out to what was referred to as General Gilke's. The hike had some severe ascents and descents as it followed alongside the Green Mountains of Vermont.

Late into the night, I found myself hiking alongside groups of racers. I bounced around from one group of people to the next, but I never attached myself to any particular group. Back at Riverside, Brian was still making his buckskin outfit as I took off into the night. I hoped that he would catch up at some point, but this was a race and I had to go. The darkness was intensified by the surrounding yellowish-white paper-like birch that peeled away from the trees and blotted out parts of the night sky and the reality that we were embarking on the paths of nature, where all sorts of animals could be lurking around. We had to be on the lookout, as a lynx, bear, or coyote could come out of nowhere. With all these thoughts about what could eat me, I was forced to wrestle feelings of fear with the reality that I was much further behind than I had wanted to be at this point in the race. From here on out, all I could focus on was pushing myself as hard as possible to catch up to the leaders. I had been competitive my entire life, and now, I was tapping into that past. I wanted to not only finish, but as a top contender.

To my surprise, someone was beating Mark Jones and this person had already returned from the next challenge. This was shocking because Mark Jones is one of the best Death Racers and one of the world's best endurance athletes. Not one to succumb to defeat so easily, I saw Mark Jones in hot pursuit of this unknown leader. At the time, I had no idea who this mysterious racer was, but he was giving Mark Jones one hell of a competition. It was exciting to see and it motivated me to push myself in hopes of catching up with those guys. Seeing that they were already returning from a challenge I hadn't reached yet made me hopeful that I was nearing it myself.

How wrong I was.

I was probably only about halfway out to General Gilke's when I approached a group of racers that were seemingly confused about where to go. There was a gate that was closed and no markers in the immediate vicinity to assure racers to cross over. This moment served me well and provided me with a chance to overtake this large group of racers. Confident in the path I was taking, even with the limited markers I had been following, I urged everyone that this was the path we had to take. I began crawling around the gate through a gap to the right of the fence where it appeared others had crossed as well. The rest followed. Continuing along the trail, I eventually saw another course marker and was reassured the path I was on would lead me to my next destination.

Not too much further along, the snowmobile trail came to an end. It was time to make a right turn onto a road that continued to add more ascents to the already arduous hike. I began to wonder whether we would venture to the same summit, Sable Mountain, that racers of that same year's Winter Death Race had to conquer in the latter half of their race. I knew that to reach that summit from Riverside it was over a 12-mile hike from working at the 2014 Winter Death Race. Based on my previous travels on this trail, I knew we had already gone far more than five miles in that direction, which increased my belief that we were headed to Sable Mountain.

As I climbed up the road, dawn began to break and another Death Race friend I had made over the years, Dan Grodinsky was on his way back from where I was headed. As he approached he stopped to take in all the natural beauty of his surroundings and the rising sun as it peaked its face out from behind the mountain tops off in the distance. As I saw him stop to "smell the roses" it snapped me out of my focused state and ushered me to exclaim to Brian, who had caught up to me, "Hold on, we have to stop and soak this all in." We stopped and turned around to do just that. Then, I saw one of the most beautiful sunrises I have ever seen. I'll always remember *that* sunrise.

Fog, mountains, and an ombré of pinks, orange, red, and blue, all fading into the most vibrant purple. The word, *"majestic"* doesn't do justice to the view that morning. The experience reaffirmed why I enjoy tackling these incredibly challenging events, they combine an unbelievable journey with extraordinary scenery.

It was soon time to snap back to reality. I was in the Death Race. If I wanted to remain competitive, I needed to hustle. I hurried down the road that seemed to continue with no end in sight until I could finally hear the sound of people, racers, working hard on the next task. As I arrived at the location of the next challenge, I was warned by some racers that the trial required a bucket. Go figure. This year, I didn't bring a bucket. Most racers didn't bring a bucket this year. Personally, I decided not to carry one because for the first time since I began Death Racing a bucket was not included on the mandatory gear list. Therefore, I assumed (unwisely) there would be buckets available if we needed them, especially since there were so many that have been left behind over the years. I should have known better! This was the Death Race, nothing would ever be handed to a racer that easily. Not without... some cost.

Since I didn't have a bucket, I slowed my pace to strategize what I could say in order to convince a fellow racer to lend me their bucket. As I approached, I saw that there was another group of racers off to the side performing some awful looking burpees. As it turned out, 1,500 burpees were the penalty that they were doling out for racers without a bucket. I've been made to complete that many burpees a few times over the years in training and probably cumulatively at both Death Races. I knew how long such a task would take. There was no way I could risk falling as far behind as that penalty would set me.

I dropped my pack off to the side of the road and walked the remaining couple hundred feet over to a man who was known at the time as notorious for creating the most challenging obstacle courses in the world. This man was known for his sadistic laugh, a man of the mountain that challenged others to redefine their comfort zone named Norm Koch. If you raced in a Spartan Race between 2013 and 2017, you probably heard the name. Norm is well known in the obstacle racing community, and he like many others started his career in organizing obstacle and endurance races by making a name for himself first as a Death Race competitor. At this time in his life, he was focused more on creating the ultimate trials of human ability. He sat there with our next array of tasks ready to be dished out to all who were willing to test themselves.

When I got to Norm he required that I grab a branch from a nearby tree. With my hunting knife secured underneath my handmade garb, it was easily accessible, and so I went straight to work serving up the man's desired branch. After, Norm instructed me to make an ax out of a rock, paracord, and any stick I could find. He showed us an example to set the expectation. From the looks of it, the quality of the craftsmanship didn't seem too important, so long as it looked like an axe was all that seemed to matter. So, I quickly fashioned any old rock I could find to a stick with my paracord and I showed it to Norm, it took all of five minutes to accomplish and I was quickly given the nod of approval. Another success.

Finally, Norm asked me if I had a bucket. I knew the penalty for not having one, and so I pretended I had one and I simply assured him that I had left it over by my bag. At this point, I had no choice but to join the rest of the racers who had made it this far and were smart enough to "play the game" and pretend to have a bucket. There was literally a line of racers who rotated the use of just a few buckets that were brought along by other racers who were kind enough to leave them behind to prevent the rest of us from failing the task. It was there, at that moment, that everyone worked together – racers against race directors. We all told the same lie so we could avoid a penalty that none of us wanted to face. Our rationale to lie to them? The bucket was never on the gear list, so why should we be penalized for not having it? This is where it's important to build bonds and connections with others, together, we would conquer what was designed to make us fail.

I waited patiently until it was finally my turn to grab one of the community buckets and head down the trail to find a stream of water that was flowing enough to fill my bucket. Everywhere I searched, I found a trickle of water at most. When I finally found something that looked like it might work, I started filling. It took a while and I remember thinking to myself that there was no way this was the stream he mentioned, but admittedly, I didn't want to continue to look.

Once my bucket was full enough I started to head back up to Norm. During my climb back up the mountainside I saw another racer heading up with a very full bucket. I quickly realized that I went further than needed and where that racer came from was the best location to fill the bucket. *"Lucky him,"* I thought. Nevertheless, I carried on and went back and showed Norm my bucket full of fresh water. I passed the test.

As I gathered my gear to continue onward it appeared that another large group of racers had showed up behind me and the others who had made it this far. Unfortunately, it seemed that they must have missed the memo about the buckets and found themselves victims of the 1,500 burpee penalty. The thing is, what they were doing did not look anything like the 1,500 burpee penalty we all feared. You see, it appeared that Norm wasn't actually paying attention to those serving their penalty, and even when he did look over, so long as they weren't just standing around he let whatever sorry excuse for a burpee they did pass.

More than half the group would stand there and perform only the jump portion of a burpee while the other half laid on the ground and pretended to do the push-ups segment, except their push-ups weren't even that, they looked more like a bunch of people lying on the ground humping and flopping their bodies around for some obscure ritual. A bizarre sight, indeed. I laughed at what I witnessed, they weren't really executing burpees, they merely faked the various segments of the burpees as a team and counted each repetition in rapid succession as if their combined effort were equated to a full burpee. As I continued to laugh at the absurdity of this race, I finished packing my gear, and took off back down the long trail to the White Barn at Riverside Farm.

On my way back, I got word that we would need our homemade axes for the next task when we would reach the White Barn. Of course, I wasn't thinking and had already ditched mine. I panicked and came to an abrupt halt and I busted out everything I needed to fashion another ax on the spot. As I returned to Riverside Farm, I was informed that I would need to have my ax examined by Peter Borden to determine how many forward rolls I would have to perform.

Upon initial inspection, Peter expressed a bit of concern about performing the first test he had lined up which was to see if the ax when swung, would and could actually do what it was intended to, split wood. Since the construction of my "ax" was flimsy at best, he casually opted to skip that test and instead he would perform a durability test. Peter took my ax and placed it in a nearby fire pit. Since the ax was made out of a stick and a rock, I figured the chances of it catching fire were quite high.

I worried. At this point, I was convinced in my mind that there was absolutely no way I would pass this test without being dealt a considerable penalty. My ax was complete garbage, I barely tried when I assembled it. At the time of assembly of this second ax, all I cared about was having one for appearances, I didn't think they would actually test them out. After a few minutes of deliberation and letting my ax sit in the fire pit, it someway somehow proved to be more resilient than any of us would have expected. It never caught fire and so without question, it passed the test!

Once again I had to gather all my gear, pack it up and head up to the top of Joe's mountain to Shrek's cabin for a quick time trial. The rules were simple: get to the top, check-in, and get back to the bottom, as fast as possible. Not knowing what we would need to do at the top, I made sure I had all my required gear but packed a little lighter on the food this time just to lighten my load. That last trek all the way out to Norm left my feet feeling a bit overworked, the short distance of this next task was welcomed.

It didn't take long to run up and down the mountain, when I returned to the White Barn in less than an hour and a half for the roundtrip, it elevated my mood and spirit. I made up a great deal of time on this roundtrip summit challenge — especially given the weight of my pack. Happiness filled my entire body. It was mid-morning and the sun was shining brightly. All that Vitamin-D had me feeling some sort of wonderful. I made my way over to the volunteers who administered the next challenge. I could see that they were handing out what appeared to be a topographical map.

As expected, it was orienteering...being that this year's theme for the Death Race was the **Year of the Explorer**, I predicted a navigational skills challenge would eventually present itself. I was right. The time had finally come.

CHAPTER 30

A RAVINE AND A CEMETERY

"The strength of the team is each individual member. The strength of each member is the team." ~ Phil Jackson

Back at Riverside, we were briefed on the next task, which could be completed in teams. I opted to wait for my friends to make their way back to the White Barn before embarking on the next challenge. All racers were given until 4 PM to successfully navigate and complete the orienteering course that they set up for us. The biggest relief of this new challenge was that we would not need to carry our full rucks for this segment of the event. It was entirely our decision what we would carry along with us, and the rest of our gear could be safely left back at our tent in basecamp. Naturally, I opted to drop my ruck and suddenly, what felt like thousands of pounds, came off my shoulders.

At long last, we had finally entered the orienteering challenge, which everyone knew we would inevitably face as a part of the **Year of the Explorer**. With items such as a compass on our gear list, many participants worried how involved and how skilled one would need to be in order to successfully complete the challenge.

When we approached the White Barn we received our

instructions for the orienteering challenge. Participants were required to collect four points in total to move on to the next challenge. Should you fail, you were done with the race. At the White Barn, we were shown a map of Pittsfield. On the map, there were points plotted with descriptors such as the Hayes Brook, the cemetery, Iron Mine, and the ravine. Some of these locations were a considerable distance to travel after all we had done, ranging from 2 miles round trip to upwards of 10 miles round trip. Picking a solid strategy was vital if you wanted to be successful at completing this challenge in the time allotted.

Each participant received a punch card, so primarily we would be looking for an orienteering hole punch at each of the locations. I observed that each hole punch had a different shape, star, moon, circle, and so forth. When I looked at the map, I quickly realized there were a few spots that I knew the exact location of the course.

First, there was the cemetery that we had just passed on our way back from Gilke's. Then, there was a ravine where I had spent plenty of time during the week I stayed in Pittsfield to help my good friend, Miguel Medina, build the foundation for what eventually became a cozy cabin in the woods built by us Death Racers. The firm understanding of the general location for both the cemetery and the ravine gave me the confidence that I would have an edge. All I needed was these two destinations on the map to earn enough points to move onto the next challenge. As far as I was concerned the hole punches shouldn't be *that* hard to find.

There was still plenty of time to complete this challenge, so I took a brief moment to collect myself. When a few of my friends showed up, I decided to team up and I reached out to Chris Rayne, Chris Accord, and Brian Edwards to tackle this challenge. The plan was to break up into two separate teams. One team, composed of those who felt the freshest on their feet, would make the long trek to the cemetery. Those two would take all of the punch cards and have them punched with the Silver Circle hole punch and then make the trek back as quickly as possible. While the two who went out to the cemetery were on their journey, the other two would climb up the ravine and locate the Green Clover hole punch wherever it was hiding. Given the location was so close to the White Barn (where we would be checking in) the assumption was it might require more time to find an item that was possibly hidden in a tree or somewhere out of sight.

Once the strategy was communicated the question remained as to who had the freshest feet? Rayne and Edwards both offered to go the distance back to the cemetery. The four of us decided to pick a spot just past an intersection on the Green Mountain Trails that led back to the stables at Riverside Farm as our meeting spot. This is where Accord and I would wait once we had located the hole punch in the ravine.

Our team split into two groups and we sought out the respective hole punch for our destination in order to maximize our points all while minimizing the likelihood of losing ourselves in the rolling Green Mountains of Vermont. With all the time I had spent over the years exploring these trails, I felt like I had become somewhat of an expert in navigating them. Specifically, I knew the fastest route to the ravine, and in my gut, I had a feeling I knew exactly where that hole punch would be hiding.

As I crossed over the rushing water that flowed down the ravine we came across the unfinished cabin in the woods. When we reached this spot, I knew it was time for us to start looking high and low. That hole punch had to be somewhere in the general area. I felt a little better now that I was moving again, so I quickly headed up the steep slope to the rear of the cabin. It felt slick and steep, but it didn't matter to me. I was determined to find the hole punch that would cut a cloverleaf into our stamp card.

The entire forest floor was covered with the beautiful colors of all the fallen leaves of seasons past. When I looked up, it was a stark contrast to the yellows and browns that covered the earth below, a sea filled with shades of green, with a dash of orange and yellow here and there danced in the wind and blotted out the blue sky. All the colors of the forest came together to make it quite difficult to identify the small green colored hole punch. Of course, the directions we were provided before leaving the

White Barn were intentionally vague. Essentially, if one was a master at finding Waldo, this was the right game for them.

I searched up and down, left and right, over and under, and slowly I found myself ascending further up this steep trail just past the cabin. Determined, I carried on and continued to scour the steep trail. After traveling a fair amount up the hillside, I turned around and shouted back to Accord to see if he had found anything. Right as my head reached the full 180-degree turnaround to look back in his direction is the exact moment when I spotted it! It was the green hole punch! I had only gone maybe 100 feet past it. There it was, down just a little way from where I stood dangling from a string that attached it to a low hanging branch. Just as soon as I had spotted our target, I alerted Chris that we were in luck. After finding this hole punch the two of us immediately began our descent to the meeting spot that our team took the time to designate before parting ways. We would now have to wait for the other two to return with the card so we could punch the second hole in it.

While Chris Accord and I waited for Brian and Chris Rayne to return, a feeling of guilt began to set in. As the sun moved across the sky and time went on, that guilt turned into a sense of remorse that developed inside of me. Did we let them down? Was it wrong of us to handle the closer, less challenging checkpoint while they went on another long hike? Why did we let them do the more laborious part? How was that fair? I started to question the logic. It still seemed sound, but I remembered I knew the area around the ravine better than anyone. I knew the most direct route there and the hope was that my knowledge would save us time locating the hole punch at the ravine. As a matter of fact, the same went for them. When they were returning from Gilke's they had spotted something purple (the same color of their hole punch) on their return trip from Norm's bucket challenge.

In my head, I justified the strategy. When they returned they would be able to go sit and relax while we went out and captured the final hole punch. Regardless of how I tried to frame the scenario in my head, the harsh reality was that Chris Accord and I definitely got the better end of the deal. To this day, I cannot thank Chris Rayne and Brian Edwards enough for going the extra mile — or, ten. Their selflessness certainly helped improve our chances of finishing, especially mine. For that, I am forever thankful.

Regardless of right or wrong, fair or unfair, it was a very efficient strategy. When Chris and Brian returned, I grabbed all of our hole punch cards from them and took off for my return to the ravine. All the rest we allowed ourselves while they made the long trek to the cemetery provided me a massive boost in my overall energy levels. The whole process of running to the ravine, punching the cards, and running back to the White Barn was quick and painless. When I returned with the holes punched, the four of us checked-in, we were one of the first few teams to finish. Our plan worked. We finished this challenge with a couple hours to spare.

Two truths were proven, knowledge (of the surrounding land and how this game works) is power, and it (sometimes) pays to win. We finished that challenge very quickly and as a result of our efforts, we earned some much appreciated rest.

CHAPTER 31

ENDLESS YOGA

"All that we are is the result of what we have thought." ~ Buddha

Having made up time with our strategy, we found ourselves beating the 4 PM cut-off by two hours. After a quick break from things, it was right back to it with the next challenge.

This time, we found ourselves back on our own as individuals. We were required to ascend to the top of Joe's mountain back to Shrek's Cabin once again. There, we would have to "start" a fire (I say that in quotes because before I took off for the summit, a little bird dropped a much-appreciated tip, I caught wind that all we needed to do was make a fire by using a bow drill).

In typical Death Race fashion, it wasn't explicitly stated that you had to use the stick and the bow drill specifically to make the fire. To be more clear, some people who were allowed to start this challenge a little earlier than us discovered that you could have a match attached to the end of your bow drill as long as the fire started. They found that there was minimal requirement to receive a passing grade for this test. With that invaluable knowledge, I made a sprint to the top with only the things I needed. As I made my way up, I received confirmation from a few others who had already made fire and were headed back. This set me up for an opportunity to make up some time if I could get it done quick enough.

When I arrived at Shrek's Cabin, I checked-in with one of the race organizers, Peter Borden, and found myself a spot off to the side of Shrek's cabin where I knew I could gather some hay from the bales that were always stashed. I quickly fashioned myself a bow drill, which is essentially a bow made from a curved stick recalling my experiences from the Survival Run in Texas. This felt like cheating knowing I was using a match to make my fire. One of the strange things about the Death Race is the lack of direct rules and instructions. With such an open box and the freedom to do anything in, around, or outside the box, it's sometimes difficult to determine what was within reasonable compromise and what was not.

I often look back on this decision and my rationale is that it was allowed, which means it was an acceptable strategy(whether it was the right strategy, is up to the person who used it). In my opinion, I feel like I cheated myself by not actually making my fire, but on the other hand, my conscience tells me that I played the "game". By playing the "game," I found myself propelling forward way ahead of the rest of the participants by doing whatever it took to complete this challenge in a smart and efficient manner within the parameters we were provided.

Here is how this challenge went down. I grabbed that bow drill that I constructed and I attached a stormproof match to the end of the drill portion of the apparatus. I then placed the strike pad on the wood notch where I needed to grind the drill into, this would normally be used to eventually generate enough friction to make fire. With my clever setup, I gave my bow drill a quick revolution back and forth and just like magic, I had a fire in an instant. Now per their instructions, I had technically just used a bow drill to create my fire. Yes, my drill just so happened to be slightly "modified", but that was part of the game. It was about listening to the instructions you were provided and finding ways to work within the often ambiguous directions given.

When I think back to past experiences at Death Races, I recall the time that another Tony rode a bike more than halfway up Joe's mountain while everyone, literally, everyone else, ran to the top. Or the time I heard some guys caught a ride to the next challenge just because they were that much more resourceful and willing to take that chance. Could they have been ejected from the event? Certainly. Were they? Nope. This prior knowledge and the wisdom of past Death Races and Death Racers' actions allowed me to easily justify my decision to manipulate this challenge in my favor. It was all a part of the "game", and I was hacking it, one challenge at a time. At other races I had participated in, the rules were a bit more concrete and something like this would never fly. Everything was open to the participant's interpretation and willingness to take a risk that could result in a penalty. Thankfully, this time, I was good to go.

By playing the game, I hacked my way through this challenge and as a result, I was in and out of Shrek's Cabin within eight minutes of my arrival. With that quick turnaround I was able to take advantage of my strong, powerful downhill running skills and navigated my way back to the White Barn at Riverside Farm in what felt like an instant.

After my return to the White Barn, myself and the rest of the racers who had come this far were directed to grab a nearby log and carry it up Tweed River Drive. With sleep deprivation setting in hard, this part of the race somewhat escapes me and the memories of it blur past, but this hike is what led me to the next challenge where we had to endure a series of tests that would span the next six, maybe seven or eight hours. At this point in the race, no one's really counting, at least I know I wasn't.

Navigating up Tweed River Drive with a log was easy compared to what came next. With this challenge, some of the hardest, most robust, athletes would suddenly break. The challenge was quite simple. It was a test administered by none other than the same mastermind who tortured me with the mile and a half log roll challenge through the goat pasture. That test was based on Special Forces training and had us rolling through each other's puke two years prior at the 2012 Death Race. This next challenge was designed and administered by none other than Jack Carry.

The test contained 26 questions with 26 matching answers. We were required to match each answer to each question using the corresponding letters. It seems simple enough in concept, right? Well, here's the thing there were a few stipulations: if you turned in your test and answered just one question incorrectly, that was it — your race was over and you would be sent on your way. Think that made it bad? It was far worse, during the entire duration of the challenge we were not allowed to speak to anyone during this test of our explorer knowledge. We couldn't overcome this obstacle via the typical Death Race style of cheating. We couldn't secretly share our answers with each other. We couldn't communicate. There was absolutely *no* talking. Pure silence.

For questions that you were unable to figure out on your own, you were allowed to wait in line where you could check whether or not one of your answers was correct each time you reached Taskmaster Jack Carry. The more questions you had the matching answer to, the easier it was to use the process of elimination in uncovering the remaining pairs until all the answers were 100% correct. The trick was that after you checked to verify one of your question and answer pairs, the challenge presented you the option to do one of two things.

First, you could elect to stand on the hillside to further work on your test to determine you had the answers. Second, you could get back in line but to do so you were required to hold a Yoga position for eight minutes at a time. Jack presented you with a few options from which you could pick your position of choice including: standing on one leg, aka tree pose, laying on your back with your feet over your head, aka dead man's pose, laying on your back while holding on to your bent legs by the feet, aka happy baby, or laying on your stomach and grabbing your ankles behind you, aka bow pose. I chose to almost always alternate between happy baby and bow pose. These two positions were phenomenal, they allowed me to loosen everything up in my back and my hamstrings. The recovery derived from this series of yoga poses was unbelievably beneficial. It was precisely the kind of self-care I needed after all the hours on my feet carrying heavy things and pushing my body to its limits and beyond. For the most part, I rather enjoyed all the long holds. The more poses I performed the more meditative the entire sequence of events became. At least, that's how I felt about the whole scenario.

The question and answer yoga madness took up hours of our time and slowly the nightfall came upon us and the cold air of the evening replaced the blistering heat of the day.

Upon our initial arrival at this challenge we were instructed to drop all of our rucks in a pile. As more racers arrived the pile grew and we were not allowed to access them. We could not grab food, or gear, or clothing or anything.

As we settled in for the evening, I found myself wishing I had been wise enough to grab an extra layer. When I first arrived, I was among one of the first groups to begin the challenge but as time passed, the line we had to wait in to ask Jack a question grew with more and more bodies filling in after each cycle. As a result of my misstep and the inability to access our rucks, I decided to do what any sensible person would after depriving themselves of sleep for more than 30 hours. I threw away all my inhibitions and started to act like a complete buffoon. I danced, I bounced, and I moved my body all around doing what I could to expend just enough energy to generate heat.

All the while I remained absolutely silent. I didn't want to risk losing my chance at redemption from the two years prior. That whole silence task was one of the most challenging aspects. It is really difficult not to want to spark a discussion when you're surrounded by so many incredible humans. What made it even worse was when someone would slip up and accidentally say or mutter a word every so often. Usually, it was the result of a race director's or volunteer's purposeful attempt to spark a conversation with a participant. More often than not, a poor soul, in their sleep-deprived state, would break their silence and acknowledge the question. In an instant their race was over.

For some participants, it was absolutely devastating. It was as though their entire world came crumbling down right then and there. To put so much effort and training into this singular event, which was much like the Super Bowl for endurance athletes. We spent enormous amounts of time and money to prepare, acquire gear, and to travel to this event. It meant everything to many of us. Getting kicked out of the event all for opening your mouth and uttering a single word was soul-crushing. My empathy felt each participant's pain. Every time a fellow racer dropped as a result of uttering a single word or peep, my heart sank. I knew how much this race meant to me, and I could easily imagine what it was like being cut for something so trivial as responding to a question.

All I could think at the time was what a shitty way this was to get cut from the race, but I had to accept the reality that this was the ultimate mental challenge. I had to keep my mouth shut or else I'd face the same twisted fate.

As the night wore on, all I could think was when would it be over. It seemed like it could go on forever. As we filled out our test and paired more questions with answers, I started to realize that some of the questions and answers were bullshit. My suspicions were confirmed when I purposefully asked a question regarding the same answer a second time and I had received two different responses each time I tried to confirm it. This was all the evidence I needed to conclude that this entire challenge was just another mindfuck, possibly one that could not be won. Immediately, I lost all of my trust in Jack. From then on I assumed he was just trying to drop people. At that point I stopped caring about the test, now it was just about enduring this madness for as long as I could. Eventually, I thought to myself, they would just shut this thing down once they dropped as many people as they needed or wanted to and they would move those who remain onto the next challenge. At least, that's what I had hoped.

Not long after my revelation, which I found myself unable to share with anyone due to the whole silence game, another racer completely lost his cool and snapped. I don't recall the exact circumstances but some of the race directors, in an effort to force participants to break their silence (I presume), opened and proceeded to dump out everyone's rucks. Mind you, when we were initially told to empty our rucks, many of us used separate dry bags within our rucks to keep things organized so even though we had to unpack those bags it would have been relatively easy to find most of our items. But they started dumping the individual dry bags and created mass chaos by mixing everyone's belongings together in one big pile.

All-in-all this was a very messed up, shitty move, one that should probably never have happened. Nonetheless, it did, and this one racer completely lost his cool. Sleep deprivation, fucking with gear, and the fact that everyone's stuff was now mixed together in this massive pile that included some participants medications was just the shitstorm we needed for the race organizers to finally bring this challenge to finality. After this racer went off on them and made a wild scene he sacrificed his bib to the raging campfire and the race directors decided it was time to move on from this to keep the flow of the race moving forward. They let everyone collect their things, and we were directed to meet at the White Barn back at Riverside Farm with no mention of how to get there. All we were told was "get to the White Barn".

Now, it was midnight the sky was dark and the disruption of all our bags made it a challenge for me to gather all of my own belongings. When I arrived at the challenge earlier, I tried to be strategic and I strung my dry bags together with a carabiner. As clever as I thought I was, I found I struggled to find half my stuff for a considerable amount of time. All the efforts I had made earlier in the race to gain a solid position closer to the front of the pack were all but lost.

After what felt like an eternity but in reality was merely five to ten minutes of frantically searching the ravaged pile, I finally found all of my race gear. By this point I had fallen far behind, I was now probably somewhere in the back half of the pack as I set out toward the White Barn. On the way down the long gravel drive that led out of that area, I saw Kristine, and I quickly realized that she had parked her rental car up there. She spent the past few hours hanging out watching all of the insanity unravel before her very eyes, while we all quietly went through each stage of the challenge. An idea popped into my head the moment I saw her. This was my chance to regain all the footing I had lost.

***

It took me two years to process this next part of the story, I struggled for a long time to come to terms with my integrity and my decision to "game the system" at this point of the race. I went through an internal struggle that forced me to do some serious soul searching.

Fortunately, on a road trip down the Oregon coast, I had a revelation and was able to talk through my hangup with my best friend who joined me. We discussed the issue I had with the decision I had made and ultimately, I came to the conclusion that what I did was the best decision I could make at that time. It was what had to be done.

***

In that moment of the race I panicked as I saw my placement slip before my very eyes, I wanted to finish this so badly and I didn't want something as stupid as this dumping of bags thing to be my demise. Not only that but, I wanted to get back to the front of the pack, where I had spent the majority of my time up until then in this year's Death Race. I recalled past Death Races and the memory of the tactics utilized by other racers to gain an edge popped into my head. This tactic was not only utilized by those who finished, but specifically by those who had in their race ranked among the top three participants. If it worked for them, surely it could work for me. It was a risk, but I was willing to do whatever it took. This was my year.

After the **Year of Betrayal** in 2012, the Death Race morphed and the attitude to finish very much became this sort of, you do whatever it takes and use a "figure it out" strategy to get there. To paint a clearer picture, if the instructions you received from a race organizer were, "get to the White Barn as fast as possible" and they made no indication in regards to HOW you must get there, it was open to interpretation as to what you would do to get there. That means, what is there to stop you from riding a bike or...in this case, hitching a ride?

Hell, if I had a jetpack, I probably could have and would have used that. The rules in the Death Race were oftentimes arbitrary. Like I said, you just have to figure out what is and what isn't acceptable through trial and error. Sometimes you could get away with gaming the system and other times you may be punished severely for taking the easy way.

In previous Death Races, I witnessed top finishers carpool their way to a challenge, and yes, there was that one time I got passed up by a finisher who was lucky enough to find a bicycle and rode all the way up Tweed River Drive to a challenge. With that knowledge floating all around in the back of my mind, I made my decision. I knew what I had to do.

Resourcefulness was a necessity and given that prior knowledge, I decided this was my moment to play the game the same way others had in the past.

Given the circumstances that surround how the Death Race worked, and truth be told, I still don't particularly feel great about this specific segment but, that's what life's all about — live and learn, right? One thing the Death Race showed me was that I was willing to take a considerable risk even though there could have been consequences. I played the risk analysis out in my head, in the Death Race, this was an acceptable strategy previously and in this moment, to me, it was worth the risk.

There was a massive risk that this could have resulted in a DNF (did not finish). Thankfully (for me), it didn't. Had I been "caught" and told that my actions were unacceptable I would have accepted my fate and walked away.

You could say, lady luck was on my side.

I caught a quick car ride with Kristine and halfway down from the top of Tweed River Drive, I jumped out of the car and ran the last quarter of a mile back to the White Barn. That one move alone saved me a solid 10-15 minutes of rucking with a 40 pound pack and provided me with the recharge I needed to prepare for the next evolution of this race.

CHAPTER 32

COMIN' IN HOT

"When I let go of what I am, I become what I might be." ~ Lao Tzu

This was where all *my* fun began.

For the next seven hours we were tasked with running as many laps up and down Joe's mountain as we possibly could. The route consisted of approximately 1,019 ft of elevation gain and about one mile of climbing that is riddled with switchbacks, out and back, for a roundtrip around two miles in length. It wasn't a short jaunt. We started at the White Barn and would take the stone stairs all the way up to Shrek's Cabin, and then run back again. This challenge was reminiscent of the challenge I helped with at the Winter Death Race that same year. There, I helped organize and photograph the event. As soon as the challenge began I recalled my experience watching it unfold at that Winter Death Race. I was standing inside Shrek's Cabin, the fire ablaze, and it was my responsibility to check participants in as they ran laps up and down Joe's snow covered Mountain. This came after they had to spend the better part of the morning dancing to Bruno Mars's hit song at the time, 'Uptown Funk.'

For some reason, as I recalled the ending of that past Winter's Death Race, the thought that this just might be the last task for the **Year of the Explorer** crept its way into my mind. At that Winter Death Race, the event concluded with racers running laps up and down the mountain. I began to ask myself, *"Could it be that this would be how they would finish this Death Race, too?"*

Could it?

Thinking back, the memory of what transpired during the next seven hours of the Death Race still gives me goosebumps to this day. This segment of the race is personally my all time favorite moment from all of my Death Race experiences be it as a participant, photographer, social media manager, or race organizer. This moment was my defining moment — where I felt the most powerful.

With a time trial serving as the next challenge, I decided to convince myself that this challenge type was the perfect way to finish off the 2014 Death Race, **Year of the Explorer**. The rules for the time trial specified that we had until 7 AM the next morning to run as many laps as we possibly could up and down Joe's Mountain. We must check in at Shrek's Cabin and at the White Barn each time. For me it could take anywhere from 25 minutes to an hour to climb this mountain depending on fatigue, pack weight, etc, the descent could be quite fast, as little as 10 minutes on a good day. Furthermore, there was a requirement of completing a minimum of five laps to pass the challenge. This was not explicitly stated but it was effectively implied. Of course, there was an opportunity for a reward dangled in front of us should we complete extra laps. Would that reward actually manifest itself, probably not but they put it out there. The best part of this challenge, we did **not** have to carry our packs.

Sweet baby Jesus, I thought to myself. The parallels to that past Winter Death Race were uncanny, I couldn't help but think that this was the time to push myself harder than ever before. This was the time to exert my maximum effort. Hopefully, this was the last thing necessary to earn that coveted finisher's skull.

Internally, I questioned whether or not I was being too hopeful.

As I made my way over to the White Barn to begin my turn at this challenge I noticed that quite a few racers had already started to ascend the mountain for their first summit. I was still a bit behind compared to where I thought I'd be given the fact that I caught a ride down part of the way. This just made me realize how badly held back from everyone else I was as a result of the whole bag fiasco.

No worries, I thought as I tried to convince myself I could catch up. Then I switched my mindset, I knew it wasn't even a question of if I could catch up, but of *when* it *would* happen. I was determined to make it so. Without the massive weight of my ruck holding me back and my legs feeling relatively fresh. I was itching to run some time trials up and down the mountain. I was stoked for the opportunity to push myself with each lap. The question switched from would I be able to catch up to, how many laps *could* I do?

I wondered for only a moment. There was no more time to think, it was time to do. I had a mission and it had already begun without me.

Without hesitation, I dropped my ruck, checked in with the staff at the White Barn and the next thing I knew I was sprinting full speed up the mountain with my destination set for Shrek's cabin. As I made the climb up the stone stairs, I noticed that some people carried their rucks. It confused me, when I checked in with the organizers I deliberately took the time to confirm whether we needed our rucks for this segment of the race or not.

Thankfully, we *didn't*.

More often than not, it pays to take the extra few seconds to confirm the rules of the challenge. This was one of those times. There I was with a massive advantage over all these racers simply because I took a little extra time to make sure I understood what was required of me. In my sleep-deprived state I didn't want to make a mistake. I was thankful that I confirmed that our objective was to run as many laps up and down the mountain as possible – all without the need for carrying a ruck.

The first ascent took me approximately 25 minutes to summit. I took no time to hesitate after I checked-in at the cabin and

I immediately whipped myself around to begin my descent. On the way down there was a massive caravan of people attempting to make the ascent. Worried I was moving too fast to avoid some of them, I began to repeatedly shout out, *"Comin' in hot, on your left, comin' in hot!"*

I repeated this like a broken record throughout the darkness of the night. The first descent took me ten minutes to complete. I checked in hastily at the White Barn where I made a quick stop at the SISU team tent for some water and one of my guilty race pleasures, a fistful of Skittles.

This process continued for the next few laps, I'd run up and down that mountain at an astonishing pace. Each lap I would check in at the top and bottom as quickly as the volunteers could get me in and out. In an effort to maximize my time on the mountain, I was careful to only stop at the team tent for a few minutes each time I came through the basecamp area. Every minute counted and I didn't want to waste any time meandering around camp. I was on a mission, I wanted to see just how far I could push myself. I wanted to see how many laps I could complete in this seven hour window of time.

By my fifth lap, I was all kinds of hopped up on Skittles and Mountain Dew. That's when Kristine forced me to stop and she force fed me a protein bar. At the time I wanted nothing but sugar, thankfully she had the sense to put me in my place. It had been hours since I'd eaten anything other than sugar and high fructose corn syrup. Like a junkie, I resisted the common sense of it all and I simply wanted more Skittles and more Mountain Dew. I was out of my right mind and she was right, I absolutely needed to consume something of more substance. Her support is something I will always be thankful for. In hindsight, it is highly-probable that I would have bonked had she not shoved that Mint Chocolate Chip Builder's Bar down my throat. At the time it wasn't what I wanted, but it was absolutely what I needed.

After that lap, my ascents had slowed dramatically, that first ascent was without question the fastest, but from that point forward each ascent after took me anywhere from five to ten minutes longer than the previous. Of course, this was expected, the more fatigued my body became, the slower my climbs would become. Oddly enough though, my descents, were an entirely different story. With each lap, my route became more precise and the way I attacked the downhill became a calculated effort. I knew all the places to accelerate and propel myself faster and faster down the mountain.

By then, I knew exactly what trees I could grab a hold of to pull and push my way downward to maximize my speed. I knew exactly what stone stairs I could bounce from to control my calculated fall down the mountain. Because that's what I was doing, I was falling. I let gravity completely take over and all I did was find a place for each foot to land as I bounced from one side to the other and back again. With each descent, my speed increased. By the time the sun began to rise, I had memorized the fastest route from Shrek's back to the White Barn, and it was as though my body floated almost effortlessly down the mountain.

On my eighth lap, when I arrived back at the White Barn I discovered I currently held the position for the most laps but my friends Mark Webb and Mark Jones were both heading back out for another lap, which would lead them to tie with me. Before that little nugget of knowledge was passed on to me, I had planned to stop. As I completed that eighth lap I thought I had done a 'job well done,' but knowing they were headed back up the mountain, my competitive edge kicked in. I wanted more. I wanted the title for most laps. I wanted to be the "King of the Mountain".

Before heading out for another lap I took a moment to evaluate how much time remained before this challenge was scheduled to be over and then I checked how long each lap had been taking me. On average, my last few ascents took close to 45 minutes and my descent took anywhere from 8-10 minutes. The climbs took progressively longer but my runs downhill were faster the more acquainted I became with the route. Given that there was just over an hour left for the challenge, I had to acknowledge the fact that if I went out for another lap by the time I returned to the White Barn I would be cutting it close to the endtime for this segment and not knowing what was next, if anything, I could be taking a massive risk.

I was determined to dominate this challenge and without much thought, I took off for another lap. I'd already far surpassed the five-lap minimum, and for all I knew I was just wasting my energy on another lap. Maybe I was being foolish, but I really wanted to clinch this challenge. As I began yet another ascent, it was clear there weren't too many people left on the mountain.

A vast majority of the racers did the minimum requirement and made the wise decision to stop after they completed the required five lap minimum. Others who hadn't yet hit the threshold continued to push to complete it while others, like myself, chased our own personal records. I chased after Mark Jones and Mark Webb even though they were both a lap behind me because something inside me told me I had to, something told me this was my moment to excel.

That final descent tested my ability to push myself beyond my perceived limitations, it showed me that even after pushing myself for nearly 48 hours that I could continue to push myself to incredible extremes and that final descent remains as one of my most fond memories from my entire Death Race experience. As the sun rose, the light glistened through the trees and lit the path which was previously only visible by the bobbing light of all the headlamps on the course. Now, my route was even more accessible to see. With a clearer path, I hopped and jumped and launched myself from one tree to another as I used my arms to propel myself down the mountain side with more and more speed. It was a strange feeling but I could almost sense that I moved faster than my previous laps.

As I made my way down I suddenly heard footsteps approaching quickly from behind. It was Mark Jones, and although I had him by a full lap, my ego couldn't help but crank up the heat. The battle was on, at least in my mind. The fact of the matter is, Mark Jones is a dominating force in the world of adventure and endurance racing. As an athlete he has been one of the top performers at many of these types of events including World's Toughest Mudder and GoRuck Selection. He is an unbelievably fast and strong human and the pitter-patter of his feet drove me to push myself even harder than I have ever pushed myself ever before.

With every lap I took almost the exact same route, making slight modifications to improve my speed of completion. With only the directions to get to the top and return to the barn, it was a challenge in which I could choose my own course. On the way up, I would take the stairs and on the way down I would take this snowmobile trail and skip a switchback section toward the lower section of the stairs. This shortcut had an extremely steep slope but it cut out a fair amount of the trail I would need to cover to return to the White Barn. As I neared the turn-off where this hidden route began, I found myself wondering if I was the only person who had been utilizing it on the descents. I soon found out as I peeled off and took my "shortcut" to the bottom that all of a sudden, the sound of Mark's feet pounding the trail dissipated. I lost him.

It wasn't until this last trip down my shortcut that it occurred to me, I was the only person who took this path to reach the White Barn. As I came to this realization, my feet began to sting with pain, I could feel my big toes burning with pain. My feet felt like they were completely destroyed. It felt as though the toenails on my big toes were disintegrating. In my head I imagined what must have been happening beneath the fabric of my shoe, I feared what I would find when I returned to the SISU tent. Even though I felt like I was losing my toenail, I pushed through the pain and ran even harder down the steep slope, I was determined to make it back in time.

As I entered the White Barn, only a few minutes remained before we had to be ready for the next challenge. Utterly wrecked from completing nine laps, I could only hope that the next challenge was nothing more than the ending ceremony. I was in shock, it turned out that my descent from the top of Shrek's Cabin to the White Barn only took me a total of six minutes.

"SIX MINUTES! Holy shit. That's so fast." I thought to myself. I felt as though I had accomplished some sort of impossible feat.

To add to my surprise, when I changed my shoes and socks, I found that my feet looked beautiful (at least by endurance racer standards) and my toenails were still intact. The pain was immense, I found it hard to believe that my toes were OK, but that last minute of running I really felt like I had just utterly destroyed them. As soon as my feet were refreshed with more Trail Toes anti-blister cream and new Injinji toe socks, my crew instructed me that I had to be in my white Tyvek suits and diaper and ready to go within the next five minutes. We also had to rinse off, so I ran over to the nearby hose and I quickly rinsed my entire body off.

Then, without even thinking twice I stripped naked right there in front of everyone, there was no time to be bashful. There was no time to think about how I could change without exposing myself. I had less than a minute left and I could not let my miraculous descent go to waste. That fact I did this without hesitation was a significant breakthrough in my self-confidence, up until that moment in time, being naked in front of others was one of my greatest fears. Up until then I was always cautious to keep myself from being seen by others, even when I was in the locker room I would take care to not expose myself to others. I was self-conscious and I didn't want others to see my goods unless they were a significant other. Given the circumstances, it was time to throw all those insecurities out the window. I had to throw away all my fucks and with that all my clothes, I had to suit up. I had to put on my diaper and my Tyvek suit and own that shit. We were all in this together, it didn't matter how dumb I looked, because we all looked absolutely ridiculous.

Once I was suited up, I grabbed my ruck, and seemingly out of nowhere I began to sob uncontrollably.

I couldn't believe the race wasn't over. All that effort. I had just wrecked myself and it suddenly felt like it was all for nothing. I let my enthusiasm and all the unbelievable high I had gotten from my sugar rush get the best of me. Additionally, I let my pride get the best of me, and now the race would continue for an undetermined amount of time. As tears rolled down my cheeks, I wondered if I left myself with enough energy in my tank to finish whatever was left to face.

CHAPTER 33

A TALE OF TWO BUSES

"Life presents many choices, the choices we make determine our future."
– Catherine Pulsifer

There I stood in a diaper and a Tyvek suit, one of those white full-body zip up suits that protects you, along with another 100 other fools. In a funny way, we were fools by choice. We signed up for this humiliation, we paid to participate in this masochistic event, and now, we stood in diapers and Tyvek suits as a collective group of fools.

With the Tyvek suit and my ruck on, I was as prepared as I'd ever be for whatever would come next. Moments before, I overcame one of my greatest fears — being naked in front of people. Conversely, I had just spent the past seven hours channeling my inner mountain goat (it felt like I had become one with that mountain). The mountain and I created a symbiotic relationship, and I found myself struggling to believe that it was me who dominated the time trial, it was me who conquered the most laps up and down that beautiful Vermont-based mountain.

The only reason I accomplished such a feat came down to sheer determination to "rest" for no more than 5-10 minutes each time I checked-in between laps. Over the course of the nine laps, my average base to summit time came out to 40 minutes and my average downhill time was a mere eight minutes with my fastest downhill time clocked in at an incredible six minutes and some odd seconds.

Was I really this powerful?

Apparently, I was.

Here's the caveat however, my unrelenting performance up and down Joe's Mountain combined with what I now consider to be my secret weapon of a diet consisting mostly of Mountain Dew and Skittles left me shattered and brought me crashing down hard at the revelation that this race was nowhere near its finality. And as a reminder that we weren't done, we were immediately subjected to a round of physical training exercises that we had to perform in unison in our Tyvek suits. My legs quivered as I was forced to hold a squat position after seven hours of quad-blasting runs up and down the mountain. My quads and hamstrings were far from thrilled. I could feel my legs shaking uncontrollably. And we were only getting started. A new day was upon us and the start of our third day at Riverside Farm meant things were about to get even more convoluted.

As it turned out we were about to embark on a journey. There were two buses waiting for us, which meant we were leaving Riverside Farm. The buses were paired side-by-side, which left all of us with a critical decision to make. One bus was yellow and consisted of cramped seats, no seat belts, and had little to no leg room for an adult. It was the kind of bus that someone who wanted to embrace that "purposeful suffering mentality" — such as a Death Racer — would take.

Definitely the right choice for a Death Racer.

Next to it was the other extreme. A luxurious coach bus complete with air conditioning, comfortable reclining seats, a bathroom, televisions, overhead storage, all the luxuries one could possibly want for a long bus ride.

When I saw the two paired side-by-side my first thought was, "It's a TRAP!"

That's all I could think when I saw the juxtaposition of these two radically different choices.

I had to think. **WWDRD?** What would a Death Racer do?

I thought to myself, There's no way I can choose the luxury coach. That's clearly the wrong choice and whoever takes that bus will without question subject themselves in their decision to some brutal form of punishment for "taking the easy way".

The time came for everyone to scramble onto the bus of their choice. A majority of the participants headed straight for the school bus. As I thought beforehand, it was the obvious choice. I just made it in time. When I had my opportunity to board the bus, I was barely able to get a seat. Of course, I was thankful that I was able to get a seat because I assumed that we would obviously be rewarded for choosing the less pleasant experience.

I thought, there was a catch, there's always a catch.

With Death Race past knowledge in mind, I had to go with my gut.

If I do this, it'll be to my benefit. It'll suck, but it'll be worth it...

I trailed off into a state of consciousness somewhere between reality and *la-la* land and within moments of leaving Riverside Farm, I found myself half asleep, yet half awake. I recall the bus circling around a parking lot up the road near the Mount Killington Ski Resort, but we never stopped. That was a surprise to me. When I saw the ski resort I was certain we would be subjected to some sort of brutal climb up the mountain or that we would have some tasks to do over there.

It would have been a great way to switch things up for the summer Death Race. I could have easily seen them direct us to get off the bus to help build an obstacle or start clearing trails or something to that effect as the Vermont Spartan Ultra Beast was just a few months away and this was the course location.

Thankfully, nothing happened at Killington.

The bus kept moving, and off I dozed once again. No matter

how hard I tried to stay awake, I just couldn't keep my eyes open. I was all out of fuel. As I closed my eyes and drifted away, I thought to myself, Where could they take us? And where did the coach bus go? What fresh new hell awaits me?

...

Moments later I awoke.

Were we back at Riverside? What's going on? Shit, how long was I asleep?!

I'm pretty sure there was some sort of instruction when we boarded the bus about not sleeping, but regardless, I had passed the fuck out. This is the type of passed out where it could have been 20 minutes or it could have been a week, and I really wouldn't have known the difference.

Whoops!

There was no time to think about that. It was time to put my game face on even though I had no clue what to expect. All I knew was that we were being shuffled off the bus and the luxury coach bus was long gone.

Questions raced through my mind, *"What would they make us do now? How long would the other group be gone, how much of a mind fuck are we about to experience?"*

It didn't matter if I wanted to finish. I had to be all in. I had to be ready to suck it up and even though I had just exerted my maximum effort on the last challenge, I had to be committed to giving this race my all. I needed to recruit every fucking ounce of energy I could muster. I could not fail. I refused.

Fortunately, I took highly-detailed notes on my iPhone during the Death Race for this last segment of the event. Directly from my notes, the words stated:

> "Bus ride to Killington aka to "New York" we went to Killington coach bus went to New York, and we went back to Riverside. Then another trip to Shrek's. Then 200 back rolls. Then off to Borden's."

When we got back to Riverside Farm, we were sent on another trip to the top of Shrek's Cabin. Thankfully, beforehand, we were allowed to remove the Tyvek suits and diapers and return to our athletic attire. As soon as I had finished yet another lap, I found myself with a total of ten laps up and down that mountain over the past 10 hours, for those of you still counting. With those ten laps complete, I probably covered a total distance over 30 miles with at least 10,000 feet of elevation gain.

Once we returned to the White Barn we were instructed to perform 200 backward rolls, of which I'm confident I bullshitted my way through. In my delirious state, I couldn't count for shit so I maybe did 100 backward rolls before I continued on my way. The truth is, at this point, it seemed like they were just killing time – and they were. My subconscious told me to stop taking the race seriously. It was time to play the game and just endure.

When we finished rolling all around the field out behind the White Barn near the Teepee, we had to hustle our way over to Peter Borden's home that was just up the trail and across the main road, Route 100. Upon receiving our directions, it was implied that the last few to arrive at Peter's would be eliminated from the Death Race. From here on out everything we did would be a matter of the survival of the fittest. I charged ahead.

All the while, I wondered, *"What are the other racers up to? They didn't really go all the way to New York, did they?"* I refused to believe that.

At this point of the event, there were 67 remaining in the race between the two buses. There were 24 who took the luxury coach and 43 who hopped aboard the school bus.

When we arrived at Peter Borden's, class was in session.

Peter's wife, Verna, was given an opportunity to join in on the fun and she turned her backyard into a school session for us Death Racers. This mostly consisted of physical fitness activities such as rolling (forward and backward), crawling on our hands and knees, leap frog races, and of course, more rolling. In a lot of ways this reminded me of a class I took in high school that was all about performing circus stunts, with the first task involving a ride on a unicycle. There were a few times I rode one of these over the course of my life, but I was anything but good at it. Nevertheless, I had hoped my decision to take that class would pay off.

We only had to ride maybe 100 feet at most. I was confident I could make that happen.

I was wrong. I failed, quickly. The tires were deliberately deflated enough to make it more difficult than it should have been on the flat grass in their backyard. I wondered if there would there be a penalty for my failure.

Next, we were instructed to make our way over to a spot where a slackline was strapped between two trees. All that was required of us was that we had to get from one side to the other. To my relief, there were no requirements to the manner in which you got across the obstacle just so long as you remained off the ground and made it from one side to the other. I was thankful that you didn't have to walk across the slackline. I knew this would be easy for me.

I decided to pretend that the slackline was much like the Tyrolean traverse obstacle that I had completed dozens of times at all the Spartan Races. The Tyrolean traverse is basically the same thing, except it's a rope that you traverse across above ground from one point to another. Normally, I can usually make it across a slackline by walking one foot in front of the other, but I am certainly no pro and this was not the time to gamble. Instead of attempting to walk across, I wisely chose to use the same technique from the Spartan Races where my belly lies flat on the rope with one leg draped over the side while the other is bent and extended and used to push my body across the rope or in this case, slackline as my arms pull me forward. In just a few seconds I was across the slackline and moving on to my next challenge at the Borden's School of Fun.

Before we could continue onto any other physical activities, we were instructed to send our family members a letter. Everyone who made it here had to take the time to pick someone they loved and cared about and we had to write them a message. Naturally, I picked my parents, they're the closest to me and have always been my driving force in all my athletic endeavors. With a quick note written to my family back home, I turned in my "assignment," and of course, I "passed" with flying colors. It was too easy. Again, this all felt like they were just wasting time.

I continued to wonder, *"How long until that bus gets back?"* My patience was tested.

After we wrote our letters home, we received our penalty for not completing the unicycle challenge, which was another 100 backward rolls. Those 100 backward rolls were immediately followed by yet another 100 forward rolls and a whole lot of crawling, hopping, and jumping our way back and forth across the yard. It was all kinds of menial physical tasks to further wear us down.

A few rounds of leapfrog later and we were broken up into teams and we had to race across the field by rolling our bodies like a log from one spot to the next. Then, our teammates would continue from there. All this rolling felt all too familiar, like the 2012 Summer Death Race — but this time with a new flavor. Little did I know, the worst was yet to come.

After all that nonsense, we were subjected to more rolling like a log. We had landscaping duty in the form of steamrolling our bodies across this brushy area. A majority of us found our bodies very itchy. Thankfully, this was followed by a submersion in the river that backed up to the Borden's residence. Once we finished steamrolling the brush we were brought down to the river and the organizers demanded that our shoulders were submerged completely under water. Until everyone was submerged up to their heads they would not start the five-minute timer. This was a group effort and the longer it took for everyone to submerge the longer the rest of us had to stay submerged. We all fell in line quickly, even those of us who didn't really want to enjoy the ice cold waters.

On that beautiful summer day in Vermont, that river water flowed with a force and we had to keep ourselves submerged for five whole minutes without popping up out of the water. Naturally, it was way more challenging than any of us had anticipated. The water was very cold, but once you got over the initial shock of the cold it was a pleasant refresher. It was a nice reset after all we had completed. My sore muscles welcomed the cold, especially all the tiny muscles in my feet. Thinking back, it felt damn good. This was probably one of the rare times that I actually enjoyed the cold water.

CHAPTER 34

THE FINAL HOURS

"By constant self-discipline and self-control, you can develop greatness of character."~ Grenville Kleiser

Once we were allowed to get out of the frigid waters, we were immediately sent back to "school". We had one last game to play before we sat down for "class time". Once everyone was gathered in the backyard, they pitted every racer against one another in an all-out race... on our hands and knees. Without putting too much effort into the race, I mostly found myself somewhere in the middle of the pack, although at times, I found myself exerting more effort than necessary. Thankfully, I didn't take it as far as some of the racers, there was a handful of racers that went so far as to tear the flesh off their knees and even the dorsum of their feet. Some racers also tore the skin off their shins, too. It looked excruciating. I only had a few scrapes, but nothing too bothersome.

After our short NASCAR-style baby crawling race, everyone was brought together to sit in the middle of the Borden's backyard. As we sat in our circle, we were taught a song complete with hand gestures. All this time it only sort of felt like we were back in school with all the random physical activities they put us through. It was truly bizarre.

The song went a little something like this, "I'm alive, I'm alert, I'm enthusiastic," and we sang this over and over all while performing gestures to go along with each line. The whole experience was ironic given most of us were barely classifiable as "alive" and we were most certainly not "alert" nor "enthusiastic." At that moment, the word enthusiastic was... well, it's an interesting description, considering how we actually felt. Most of the racers were far from enthusiastic with sleep deprivation factoring in, but some Death Racers had a reverse effect from the sleep deprivation and in a way appeared "enthusiastic" and "slap-happy." Sleep deprivation can be like a wild card, you never know what version of yourself you'll get.

Once the "alive, alert, enthusiastic" game came to its highly-appreciated end, we 'graduated' and were instructed to collect our gear and belongings before being sent back out into the wild for our next challenge. All the while, I still couldn't help but think they were just putting us all through the paces to kill time while we waited for the other bus to make a round-trip to New York. From Vermont, it's a minimum of a five-hour drive to New York, so the round-trip would take at least ten hours, plus however long they would spend doing whatever it is they would be subjected to while still dressed in their diapers and tyvek suits. I found it unbelievable that they would divide our race experiences so dramatically.

To keep us occupied for the next task, we were to re-enter the river at the same spot where we dunked ourselves shoulders-deep earlier and we had to trudge up river to the home of Marion Abrams, the lady behind the camera for all things Peak Races. It was our mission to provide Marion with some good ol' fashion "volunteer" Death Race style community service in the form of manual labor. While some loathed these tasked, I really loved directly giving back to the local community and everyone involved in putting these incredible life-changing experiences together. They opened up their homes and land to give us a place to develop a deeper connection with ourselves, others, and nature. Our efforts at Marion's residence would have a direct impact on her and her family's ability to protect their home from a river known to rise quite high after the snow melts.

THE FINAL HOURS

Over the next few hours, we gathered boulders out of the riverbed and orchestrated a rhythm for production as we collectively alternated between gathering and stacking. Together we utilized our human-generated power to manufacture an outstanding retaining wall that could act as a blockade to prevent flooding the next time the river rose to levels beyond the norm. The most challenging part of a task like this stems from the slick nature of the riverbed rocks. It was paramount that no one twisted an ankle. We had come so far and to do such a thing would be devastating to anyone's chance to finish.

After we successfully completed the task – a victory for us – we were gathered by Johnny Waite and given some relief. We had five minutes to eat, drink and go to the bathroom. While this was a nice reprieve from everything else we'd been subjected to since boarding that yellow bus, it was still quite the challenge to overcome when you feel a need to complete all three needs in such a short timeframe. Once we finished taking care of all of our basic "input" and "output" needs we were instructed to gather our packs and we were blessed with 20 minutes of rest. The only catch... we were not allowed to move, not one bit.

We were allowed to position ourselves however we wanted, but once we found our position we were not to move for the next 20 minutes. I chose to lay my pack down against a log. I propped my body up in a half sitting, half laying down position, my legs extended out in front of me with my torso at a 45-degree angle resting my weight against my bag and the log behind it.

Although that doesn't sound so bad for a Death Race, it's important to remember that we were not allowed to sleep or move a muscle. To earn this rest, we had to find a position and hold that position. Most importantly, our eyes must remain open. This was not an opportunity to sleep, it was an opportunity to rest.

At this point more than 50-hours had elapsed. To be given the chance to lay down and not sleep was a sick and twisted trap in waiting. The Race Directors found a way to provide us with this very relaxing moment while still maintaining their sadistic methods to continue to deploy a different kind of suffering. I wondered if the Race Directors were purposefully incorporating a variety of tasks that ultimately aided us in our journey. Thinking back on the day's numerous tasks there had already been a few beneficial tasks in just the past few hours.

First, they allowed us a period in the river that actually gave our bodies a much needed "ice bath", which is known to aid in recovery. Now here we were lying down, resting our bodies, and we were allowed a chance to meditate.

As I lay there meditating I couldn't help but wonder, would they cut us if we fell off into a dreamland? Could something as simple as falling asleep be the end of another Death Race journey?

I hoped not, just as I began to feel the heavy weight of my eyelids.

My eyes gazed up into the deep blue Vermont sky and I thought, this feels like the most difficult challenge yet. How am I supposed to lie here wide-eyed, unflinching, and then I remembered the song we were taught at "school" an hour earlier, *"I'm alive, I'm alert,"* and hopefully once we were allowed to stand back up, *"I'll still be enthusiastic."*

I noticed there was some self-doubt creeping its ugly head in, but I refused to let it. I had to be enthusiastic when I was done with this meditation. If I wasn't, the thought of finishing would be impossible.

That's when I remembered the importance of smiling, of being thankful for what I'd already accomplished. Suddenly, I felt a heightened sense of just how alive I really was in that moment. That feeling in that meditative state made it possible to instantly appreciate the present, everything in the here and now, who I was, who I had been, and who I was becoming.

I discovered what it meant to be present, to be truly aware. In that moment, I found my happy. I found myself fully *alive*.

I repeated in my head, "don't fall asleep... don't... fall... don't fall... asleep..." try as I might I could feel myself slowly starting to drift away. The hours and hours of work were compounding. I was losing my ability to maintain control of myself. I thought to myself, I can't let this happen again, I had already fallen asleep on the bus when we weren't supposed to and nothing happened then but that moment had no attachment to this moment. If they wanted to punish us for falling asleep, they could and would. I fought back against my mind and my body's desire to fall asleep by blinking my eyes with intentionality.

Suddenly, I vaguely heard the soft sound of Johnny Waite's voice whispering subtle instructions to those of us who had yet to fall fast asleep. As it turned out, I wasn't the only one struggling to stay awake.

He softly spoke a few directions to the lot of us, "Okay everyone, in a minute I'm going to tell all of you to get up, those of you that can hear me get up quietly, and do not let the others hear you. Gather your belongings, then head back upstream."

The rest period was over. Those of us who were still conscious slowly collected our packs and strapped them back on before we made our way quietly back into the river. Nearly half of the racers were unreservedly passed out, and they had not a clue that we were evacuating the area. It didn't take long though for them to snap out of their slumber, unfortunately for some, it was already far too late. Because they dozed off they would be far enough behind to find themselves trailing and falling into the danger zone. As I expected would happen, we heard the announcement, "The last five back to Borden's are out." The speed of movement across the entire flock of Death Racers intensified all around me. It was a treacherous sprint across the rocky riverbed. I tried to maintain my balance as I hustled from one slippery rock to the next. It felt extremely dangerous. One small fault in my movement on this slick surface and I could easily snap an ankle. I moved with cautious haste.

When I scurried my way up the river back to the embankment where we first entered the water, I emerged just as quickly as I had entered and returned to Peter Borden's backyard. I sat down and awaited our next set of instructions. A massive wave of relief swept over me as I realized I once again managed to maintain my position. I was still in this. Minutes later, five more were "sent off the island."

There was no hesitation from the race organizers to send them packing. It was unbelievable to me and I started to wonder if I had picked the wrong bus. Considering how long the drive to New York would take, the other guys and gals probably arrived in New York a couple hours ago. That whole time they were riding that bus, here we were busting our asses for hours with multiple cuts to the remaining participant count. Still elated that I was in it, I couldn't help but wonder what other wicked games would await.

It wouldn't take long before we would find out.

Log Rolls.

Motherfuckin' log rolls. Suddenly, it felt as though I was reliving the 2012 Death Race all over again. I feared I would find myself puking my guts out all over the place, again. Upon hearing this I remember thinking to myself that this was just wonderful. It didn't matter though, I didn't have time to care about what this meant. In my mind and in my heart nothing could or would stop me from finishing this Death Race.

I swallowed my fear and I got down on the ground, laid my body flat on the ground, and I rolled. Thankfully, it wasn't a repeat of the 2012 Death Race where we rolled a quarter mile loop six times to completion. This year, all that was required of us was to log roll the perimeter of the yard just one time. It was nothing compared to the challenge two years prior and to say I was thankful this log rolling experience wasn't anywhere near as long nor as vomit-inducing as the **Year of Betrayal** would be a massive understatement.

As soon as we finished rolling, we sat at attention with our packs in front of us and we waited until we were instructed to make haste for Riverside Farm. Once again, the last five would be ejected from the race. The more and more these eliminations continued the more battleworn we all became, it was every man and woman for his or herself. With a fully weighted ruck strapped tightly to my back, I sprinted up the driveway and out onto Route 100 heading back to the White Barn where it all began some 56 hours ago.

CHAPTER 35

SKULLS

"There is only one success – to be able to spend your life in your own way."~ Christopher Morley

In the heat of the day, I barely knew which way was up and which way was down. What should have been running became more of hobble as I shifted the weight of my pack back and forth to move with some sense of purpose. As I approached the White Barn along with a few other racers, we were immediately directed to drop our bags and run over to grab a cement bag. The moment was chaotic — a flurry of events unraveling in what seemed to take place all within a single heartbeat.

As the remaining Death Racers made their arrival at the White Barn, another round of cuts began and once again, the last five were sent on their way. Suddenly, it was very apparent that the field had dropped some 20-30 participants since we boarded the buses all those hours ago. Those who remained were battling one another as if it were for their life — a friend you were running next to was also the competition — the difference between making the cut and going home all boiled down to who wanted it more.

At this stage, it was every racer for themselves. You had to give it your all if you wanted it all. I wanted this Death Race more than anything. I wanted to finish what I started all those years ago when I first saw some online advertisement for this crazy thing called the Death Race.

It all started with me questioning whether I had what it took to conquer the Death Race or not, and through the process of answering that question I subjected myself to a multi-year endeavor that required the Courage to start, the Power to overcome, and the Wisdom to learn from my mistakes and successes to finally overcome all the trials these masters of suffering, better known as the Race Directors, conjured in an orchestrated effort to make us quit. Many would find any excuse they could hold on to and believe in to make the tough decision to give up, while others dug deep within and found the courage, power, and wisdom to ask themselves to do whatever it would take to walk away with a skull.

As for myself? I wanted that skull.

I wanted to know I had it all.

I wanted to know if I could survive anything this race would throw my way.

I wanted to believe that if I could finish this, that it meant I could succeed at all the trials and tribulations that life may hold.

I wanted to finish the Death Race.

I wanted to do it without that "unofficial" tag.

I wanted to outsmart the creators of an event considered by publications around the world among the top 10 ultimate endurance-based sufferfests, and this was *my* year.

This year I was more relentless than ever before. Over the course of the past 58 hours, I had given a massive effort not only to do whatever it took to finish, but to do what it took to perform, to excel, and to give it my all.

In all the chaos, I had a flurry of thoughts ranging from how much more I wanted to push, to how broken I actually felt. Though my body began to feel broken, my mind remained sharp. In an instant, the weight on my shoulders came crashing down. My cement bag exploded almost as soon as I collected myself and positioned myself with it held overhead as directed. Quickly, someone stepped in as my hero (in all the chaos I can't recall who) and provided me with me with a sizeable black contractor's bag.

As soon as I had it opened, I frantically tried to get ALL the cement powder back in there. I feared my bag wouldn't weigh in properly when I made it to wherever it was we had to go with these 50-pound bags of cement. That sudden realization caused me to panic, I was utterly overwhelmed by what had just happened. Thoughts about how far we had come flooded my mind and tears began to roll uncontrollably down the dirt-ridden skin of my cheeks.

I knew deep down I couldn't let this bag of cement lead to my demise, there was no way I could give up. I had come too far.

With all my experience, this felt like it was the smoothest personal participation I had in this masochistic race. My past years engaging as a participant, in media development, and as an organizer, cultivated myself into a wise and powerful Death Racer.

My time was now.

Through my tears, I found the power within to self-motivate and carry on.

The old adage of putting one foot in front of the other was all it would take. I knew if I just kept moving forward, it would guarantee my success. That's all I needed to do, keep moving forward.

With my 50-pound cement bag, I was sent with the remaining racers on a trek to the infamous ravine that lead up to what I know as Miguel's cabin, but is commonly referred to as the Crack Shack. We had to ascend that wonderfully-terrifying terrain while keeping our cement bags fully intact.

"*Lovely,*" I thought to myself.

At first, my bag felt surprisingly light. However, it didn't take long to fatigue and after a few hundred steps, I could really feel the weight on my shoulders. Throughout this challenge I found it bizarre how in one moment I could barely notice the weight and then suddenly, it would feel as though I was about to collapse. The first half mile or so from the White Barn to the entrance of the ravine was mostly flat, but once we entered the gorge, the intensity increased in correlation with the incline. The ravine was treacherous and the rest of the surrounding terrain was wicked slick. As the water flowed down this ravine it pooled in some areas and flowed in others. I traversed up and over rocks, fallen trees, solid roots, the whole while I focused on keeping my bag of cement high and dry.

As I slogged my way further up the ravine, I found the terrain became less forgiving. That route was less than ideal. The most humorous thing was knowing that just a few feet higher up there was a perfectly good trail that could have been used to carry the cement bag up, but that'd be too easy and not very Death Race-like and I was certain there were volunteers or organizers watching to make sure we stayed in the ravine.

WHAM!

I slipped. As I attempted to climb up a series of fallen trees, roots, and whatever else it was that supported these pseudo steps in this ravine, I fell forward and the cement bag parted my neck and formed two sacks that smacked me on both sides of my face. *BAM!* I felt trapped. For a moment I found myself stuck between two 25-pound sacks of cement. With my head held down I laid there on the log just in front of me.

With my head pressed down onto the log I felt helpless if only for a moment. I didn't feel entirely defeated but I was damn close. With tears of rage, I grunted and groaned and dug deep into my soul to muster up all the might I had left. I picked up my head along with the two 25-pound sacks of cement that forced my face to press into the log beneath me and I hoisted them up from the ground. I recovered to a vertical position and took a moment to sit on the trunk. I needed a moment.

"Ahhhh ...sweet relief," I thought to myself as I let everything go.

I held nothing back and I pissed myself... right then and there as I rested on the same log I had just made face-to-face contact with, I pissed myself. I couldn't move, I couldn't hold it, and I didn't even think about it, it just happened. I had reached my limits – it was a 100% no-fucks-given kind of moment. I just pissed myself and suddenly, I didn't give a fuck how much the cement bags weighed or how much they sucked. I didn't give a fuck that I was emotional, I didn't give a fuck that I was alone in that ravine. At that point, I remembered that I had been forging myself to become unbreakable. I remembered I had everything I needed within me to finish the race. I just had to stand up and carry-on. That's all I had to do... stand up, carry that cement bag and continue to navigate my way up the ravine. I would NOT stop until I was told that I finished the Death Race.

And that's just what I did. I lifted myself up, I laughed off the fact I just pissed myself and I continued on my way up the ravine. I carried that bag up until I finally reached Norm. He stood there grimacing at me as I struggled with my cement bag. He stood in front of the cabin that was erected on the foundation that my friend Miguel and I had worked on a year and a half prior. Norm stood there knowing full well I had lost some of my cement powder when we all stood by the White Barn earlier. He saw what happened and now here he was checking our cement bags at the checkpoint.

In that instant, a wave of fear swept over me. I dreaded what was about to happen. I had no idea what he had planned for us and as far as I knew, he had the power to do whatever he wanted. Would he let me pass or would he end it all for me?

Next to Norm there was a plank that sat on a balance point to create a scale. On one end, he had what was presumably the expected weight to match our cement bags and on the other an empty space where he quickly directed me to place my bag. He laughed his happy ass off the entire time with this twisted grimace. He knew I wouldn't have the proper weight.

"Would he let me pass, or was I screwed?" I continued to wonder as I approached the scale.

My bag didn't quite balance the scale out. Though, it wasn't off by much, there was enough weight that the scale teetered and never quite reached perfect harmony. I looked to Norm. He laughed again and he directed me to place my bag in the pile next to the others and to get out of there.

"That was it, I was home free!" I thought to myself.

I took off, elated, as I made my way back to Riverside Farm.

"What's next?" I eagerly wondered.

Was this really the last task? Or how much more did we have to do? And when the hell was that other bus coming back?

These questions raced through my head as I made my way back down the trail that skirted alongside the ravine I had just successfully navigated with nearly 50-lbs of cement.

My mind continued to race. Without question, this was one of the hardest Death Races I had witnessed or participated in as we closed in on 60 hours elapsed time into the relentless pursuit to reach a finish line that didn't even physically exist.

That's what I signed up for, a race that had no defined start and no clear finish. That was what made the Death Race so special. It was a race designed in a way that is reminiscent of life, you don't know when it starts, just like you have no choice how your life begins, you're just born one day, and the harsh reality is you don't know when it will end either, the lights go out, and just like life we all must find our own path from start to finish.

Once I made it back to Riverside, the lot of us were not allowed to leave the perimeter of the horse corral outside the White Barn. The consequence for doing so would be immediate ejection from the race. Once everyone had completed the cement carry and made it back, we were informed that we would not be allowed to leave the corral for the next six hours. That was it, that was all we had to do. Stay behind a wooden fence line for six hours and we would finish the Death Race. Of course, feeling skeptical many of us wondered what else was in store.

During our time in the corral, any racer's crew members were forced to leave the corral and could only talk to us from the other side of the fence. In a way it resembled a sort of jail.

Thankfully, the fence was your standard stable fence, which consisted of a post every six feet and a couple of rails that were parallel to each other no more than three or four feet off the ground. To keep me company, Kristine set herself up alongside the fence and made an area to rest while we all waited for the other bus to return from New York.

Time went by and we all kind of bounced around, shared stories from the weekend and revelled in all we accomplished. At one point, the race staff made a deliberate effort to remind us that everyone on the New York-bound bus still had their diapers on and that we should be very kind and considerate to every one of them upon their return.

It was hard to comprehend with the lack of sleep but it would seem we were being told that essentially the entire bus spent their day in New York unable to use the restroom.

I couldn't imagine what I would do in that situation other than unrealistically hope that I wouldn't need to expel any bodily waste throughout the day.

The thought of how pungent the smell everyone on that bus must have been subjected to haunted me for the remaining hours in wait.

After that information was divulged and a few hours had passed, we were all thoroughly convinced that we received the better end of the deal. Even though our bus involved time hacks, and tons of manual labor, the thought that we didn't have to spend a day in a diaper filled with our own secretions, made us all feel better about our choice in bus. I was thrilled that I selected the yellow bus. It seemed as though our deal far surpassed the mild luxury afforded by taking the coach bus. I just couldn't imagine what sitting in my own poop for five hours on a bus would be like, all in an effort to finish a race to earn a simple plastic skull. It seemed beyond demoralizing, it seemed outright disgusting, and was easily the cruelest thing any of these absurd endurance events could subject a group of people to do in order to earn a finish.

My disgust turned to anger as I thought about the circumstances. *"What the hell was wrong with them? Would they really do this to a group of people?"* In my head I asked dozens of these questions. It just didn't seem right. It was so incredibly wrong.

At the time, my brain was quite exhausted from all we had endured and as outrageous as it all seemed, I was convinced that it wasn't entirely impossible. I wasn't sure if it was right, and I wasn't willing to rule out the possibility.

After six long hours of killing time, making multiple attempts to nap, and spending quality time with my fellow racers, volunteers, and anyone who wanted to talk about life outside the Death Race, we finally received word that the other bus was about to arrive. Again, we were reminded not to treat the racers in any particular way, the organizers emphasized that they had been through a lot. I remember it was kind of awkward to hear this, once again I thought to myself, this just didn't seem right, would these people really do such an awful thing to their fellow humans?

Of course, they wouldn't. And, how could we be so gullible? Many of us were convinced that this was the reality, our comrades who took the luxurious bus just rode back from New York City sitting in diapers filled with shit. There was no way that could actually be true. Or could it? I didn't really know.

Thankfully, when the bus arrived, and everyone unloaded, we all promptly realized that the other racers had not been subjected to such cruelty. Once the group of racers made their way off the bus, everyone was gathered around and speeches of empowerment, betterment, and encouragement were set in motion and we were told to take what we learned here at this event and to go out and make our own impact on the world. It was our turn to make a difference in the world by taking what we learned from this event and sharing it with our fellow humans.

We had done something, as Don so eloquently put it. Now it was time to *DO something*.

By signing up, showing up, and participating in one of the grittiest races on the planet, we had seen what it means to be alive. We tasted what it was like to suffer, to work through our most primal instincts, to have all of life's modern luxuries stripped away, in this we learned what it means to give it our all and to never give up regardless of the circumstance or the obstacle. People will challenge you daily and you are going to be faced with a myriad of challenges that can make you want to quit, but after going through something like this, it is almost as though you transcend the minor difficulties life presents to you on a daily basis. Things that bother most people become trivial to someone who has overcome such adversity.

It doesn't have to be the Death Race, there are plenty of trials out there that test your grit and forge you into a hardened, more resilient human being. Whether you find it in doing hard labor or you discover it summiting mountains, or by sailing across the sea, running across the desert, there are many ways to achieve this heightened state of existence. After this experience I recommend to search for your own Death Race, whatever that may be.

Find it, work at it, and overcome all the obstacles you'll face along the way through trial and error and make yourself become whatever it is you want to be. You have it in you to persevere and to become who and what you want.

To succeed in any endeavor, you must have the Courage to start. You must be courageous and try the things that intrigue and interest you. And you can't give up when things don't come easy, or when they don't go your way. If you really want to be an artist, a musician, a programmer, or whatever it is, you have to dig deep and have the courage to start, over and over. I encourage you to chase after the goals that you know will make you a better version of yourself. Go and do this with unabashed enthusiasm.

Once you've found the courage to start, you must develop the Power to conquer whatever your challenge is. By power, I don't necessarily mean strength, but your ability in whatever skillsets are required to master your challenge. Whatever skills or technique is required to be developed, whatever it is, you need to build the power to succeed. You need this power so you can push through the struggles and the trials you are sure to face in your endeavor to succeed. Power is what it takes to overcome all the obstacles we inevitably will face.

You can't conquer life with courage and power alone, however. The last piece of the puzzle takes a little bit longer to develop, it's the Wisdom you gain from all your trials, from your failures and your successes. It's this wisdom you develop that you need to conquer the obstacles you'll face on your road to success. Wisdom only comes about from having the courage to start however. You can't gain wisdom without starting. Once you get started, your actions will help you to develop the power to continue moving forward in the direction you wish your life to take you. Once those two are set in motion, if you keep your mind open to it, and you take the time to learn from your mistakes, and you don't give up, even when your head is metaphorically smashed between two 25-pound sacks of cement, only then, will you have what you need to develop the wisdom to succeed. With the courage to start, the power to conquer, and the wisdom to overcome, you can achieve anything you set your mind to. You have it in you to be what you want to be, it just takes, courage, power, and wisdom to get there.

And so, my journey had finally come to an end.

It was all over.

After three long years of trial and error, I had finally done it.

Over 66 hours into my third attempt at this thing called the Death Race, I found myself standing among the few who had what it took to start and finish the 2014 Death Race. To explain how I felt is difficult. It took nearly everything I could find within me to overcome the massive challenge I had set out to conquer four years prior.

Through my courage, power, and all the wisdom I developed along the way, I finally got what I came for. After four years of analyzing, and methodically dissecting the inner workings of this race from the inside out, I had finally done what I set out to do, I finished. In those years, I lived it, breathed it, and studied every aspect of it. I observed and analyzed the race in all its variations, the Mexico Death Race, the Winter Death Race, and the Team Death Race, during this time I even helped lead segments of them. With all the knowledge and all the power I developed over the years, this was the culmination of a multi-year journey. I had finally figured it out. Because of my relentless pursuit to earn a Death Race skull, I emerged as one of the victorious.

A Death Race Finisher.

Not unofficial, or any of that ambiguous nonsense.

Simply, **Finisher**.

It felt damn good, and even all these years later, it still feels good. The Death Race is and will remain a pivotal period of my life. It showed me who I really am, it allowed me a chance to face my demons head on, and through all the highs and lows, the pain and suffering, it became clear, the only way to succeed at this race, and at life, is to keep on keeping on. To persevere through even the darkest moments, to know that things can and will always get better, you just can't give up. You have to fight through the dark, to see the light. This race showed me who I am, it gave me a new frame of reference on how I can live this life, my life, to the fullest. The more I push myself, the more I challenge myself to grow, the more exciting my life can and will be. This race showed me what can happen when you keep forging ahead, and when you never give up on your dreams.

With that said, I'll leave you with this old adage for whatever your Death Race is, if a first you don't succeed, try, try again. Then, try again, and maybe you will fail, maybe not. If you do fail, don't think of it as a failure, realize that it's a moment to learn. Take the time to learn from your mistakes and then go try once again. And if you fail still, perhaps you continue to learn something new with each failure. Life isn't always going to allow you to figure everything out on your first go. Sometimes you must try, try again. And that's okay. That's how you conquer life. You keep trying. You keep improving. You keep learning. You keep doing.

Now, go find your "Death Race" and start your own legend.

The End.

EPILOGUE

After the Death Race, life became easier to handle. I learned a lot in the three years chasing my spot among those capable of finishing a race with a less than 20% finisher rate. In those three years of competing, I discovered the importance of teamwork and what it really means to think outside the box. We hear that phrase all the time, but at the Death Race, you really find yourself exposed to challenges that force you to get creative. You either get creative or you fail.

The Death Race is designed to find your weaknesses, expose them, and make you fail. Whenever I was smiling, I was invincible. It's really hard to defeat someone who is confident in themselves and believes in themselves. It took a lot of Courage to show up to the Death Race each and every year. That's why it is one of the principles and virtues I focus on in this book. Courage is one of the most critical virtues for anyone who wants to have a more adventurous and fulfilling life. Courage is what it takes to try the new thing you keep telling your best friend about, and doing it with or without them. Courage is the ability to do something that frightens you. We must have courage if we are ever going to succeed at materializing our dreams. It was my dream to complete this race deemed one of the top 10 most difficult events on the planet. To do that, I needed the courage to start. I had to sign up, pay the $400+ entry fee, collect all the gear, buy the plane ticket, train my ass off, and show up ready to endure whatever was thrown my way.

Once I had that goal, it was all about maintaining that courage and using that to develop the power to overcome all that I would face along the way. I did that through deliberate immersion in the culture and training required to succeed. In 2011, I spent hours training every day after work to begin this journey. Sometimes, I even trained before work as well. On weekends, I hiked with a weighted ruck through dense forests in Illinois all through the night to acquaint myself with the grit required to endure a night, alone, in the dark. In front of my parent's house in the suburbs of Illinois, I flipped tires, then ran up and down the stairs of their two story home. Every day, I focused on one thing, the Death Race. My power wasn't developed overnight, heck the first year I went into the race injured, which I don't recommend. And yet by 2014 I was fully recovered from my shoulder surgery, full of strength and had developed a gusto for suffering. I made the art of suffering my passion and learned that succeeding at this event, or any of life's endeavors, requires hard work, dedication, focus, and consistency. That's how you develop power.

Being strong and mighty isn't everything though, you have to be smart to finish a Death Race. When it comes to brain vs. brawn, I don't want one or the other, I want both, always. Developing your wisdom in an area requires a relentless pursuit even when you falter. I took note of my mistakes, the mistakes of others, and I analyzed the race from a variety of angles. I put myself out there, wrote about my experience, digested my feelings and emotions, and thought about how I could better prepare and succeed with each Death Race. Through dedicated, persistent, trials of success and error, I effectively enhanced my knowledge in what is required, permissible, and applauded in the Death Race, and in doing so found myself with the wisdom necessary to finish the event.

These three virtues, **Courage**, **Power**, and **Wisdom** are what I believe it takes to conquer all of life's obstacles.

When we put ourselves in the face of adversity, we learn how to become more resilient. The more resilient we are, the more likely we are to survive — whatever it is we need to survive. Life is full of obstacles, some more unforgiving than others. Developing a form of obstacle immunity, through the purposeful subjection of oneself to manufactured adversity, allows you to become more unbreakable.

To this day, I still believe and practice this. While I don't subject myself to as many events as I used to, I still get out of my comfort zone constantly with things like mountaineering, backcountry camping, and other outdoor endeavors, but also, singing karaoke, learning to play the saxophone, attempting to learn some basic Kanji, Japanese, and Mandarin. When it comes to getting out of your comfort zone, all around you there are opportunities to do so. At work, at home, with how you approach friendships, personal development, and social activity, life is full of chances to be courageous, to become powerful, and to be wise. Find your niche, and make your own magic. This life is yours, and it's up to you how you spend it. Safe and sound, or ready for adventure.

ACKNOWLEDGMENTS

When people say something is a labor of love, it signifies the significant amount of effort they poured into it. For me, this book was very much a labor of love, over eight years in the making and it has finally come to a close. As I look back on all these years, it's clear to see there are a great many thank you's that need to go around. I must preface these acknowledgments with the reality that I may forget some; it's not because what you did didn't matter. It is just that a lot of time that has past along the way, and I may not remember every single person who contributed to my Death Race experience. There's so damn many of you. So to all of you who have lent me a hand along the way, I thank you, sincerely.

Above all else, I want to extend a massive thank you to my parents for birthing me, raising me, challenging me, and supporting me in all my endeavors. Darnell and Rich Matesi have been instrumental in shaping me into the human I am today, and for that, I am forever thankful. While we don't always agree, I appreciate how much you challenge me to be the best version of myself, always. You two are the best kind of parents there are. This world would be a better place if there were more parents like you in it.

My little sis, Mariah, you've put up with a lot growing up with a brother like me. Thankfully, you've always been a great part of my support system; I love you, kiddo. I can't thank you enough for always listening to me, even when I'm rambling. I can't wait to have more adventures with you. I love you.

Thank you, Chad Weberg, you're at the top of my list because if it weren't for your support after that first Death Race, I don't know how easily I could have found myself where I am today. You broke down a whole lot of barriers for me, and for that, I am forever grateful.

Joe De Sena, obviously, for putting up with my countless emails, frequent drop-ins to your farm in Vermont, and for all you have done to help me move my career forward and teach me some critical leadership skills along the way. I cannot thank you enough for what you are doing for this world. You are ripping people off the couch, getting them out of their comfort zone, helping them overcome PTSD, providing them with substance abuse help, and taking in those who need that extra push to overcome their weight challenges. You are the kind of leader who does so by example. You are a one-of-a-kind human, and you are making a massive impact on this planet. Keep it up.

Andy Weinberg, for the role you played in developing this event in its early days and helping me out when I was unable to afford the high cost of registration my second year.

Daren de Heras for always being there for me during these insane challenges we have put ourselves through over the years. Meeting you has been one of the greatest blessings. I'm looking forward to many more adventures with you, ol' man. ;-)

Team SISU and everyone who is a part of it, you guys and gals have supported me through a lot of these endeavors, and for that, I am forever thankful.

Mark Webb, for always being my Death Race buddy, for picking me up from the airport and giving me a place to stay. You were always there for me, like the big brother I never had. I am so thankful I had the opportunity to race with you and to get to know you and your son Xander over the years. It's been wonderful having you be a part of my life.

Andé Wegner, you became like a sister to me over these past

few years of endurance racing, I can't thank you enough for always being there for me. You've done so much.

Kristine Iotte, you helped me through my last Death Race; for that, I cannot thank you enough.

Morgan McKay, you were the person who helped me carry-on at that first Death Race in 2012, you were there through the good and the bad, and together we came out the other side as better versions of ourselves. Thank you for all the good times on those trails in Vermont.

Matt B. Davis, we've been through a lot, and you have been there since that first Death Race. Having me as your very first guest on your podcast is a memory I'll treasure always. Thanks for being there. Thanks for cheering me on. Thanks for being a friend.

Johnny Waite, the man with more wisdom and more love than anyone else I've ever met. From the moment I met Johnny, I knew he was a magical kind of human being, the kind who has seen some shit, and yet he always smiles and always finds the good in situations. I value our friendship and the many lessons you've given me along the way. Thank you for pouring so much love out into the world.

Rob Barger, it's been an immense pleasure getting to know you over all these years and racing with you. Thanks for all your tv, movies, and music references out on course, they always bring a smile to my face.

Amelia Boone, you're one badass woman, it was an honor to train with you for that first Death Race. I'm still quite fond of the moment in the woods when you told me you had yet to swing an ax. Now I look at you, all these years later and you've become one of the most iconic females in obstacle and endurance racing. Thanks for being there to join me on this journey so early on.

Jon Townsend, more than anyone else for putting up with all my requests to edit my blog posts, look over my work, and to help me edit this entire book multiple times, you are the kind of friend that is so rare to find in this world. I am so thankful that we connected back in high school and have since maintained this friendship of ours. I can only hope it continues to grow and flourish. We still have unicorns to ride.

Erinn Carlson, though your assistance came long after my Death Race years, your support, encouragement, and motivation helped fuel me to see this book through to completion. Without your countless hours pouring over the pages of this book, the first edition of this book would have bared many typos and comma-splices (my arch-nemesis in writing). Thank you for all you have done to help me turn this book into the refined work it has become. You are my rock.

There are many many others for whom I could thank, but to continue would be like writing another book, so if you've helped me along the way, know that I thank you from the bottom of my heart, I will cherish the crossing of our paths now and forever. Thank you, everyone, who made this journey possible. I love all of you.

GLOSSARY

Amee Farm - A Farm that is located by the Amee Farm Lodge as well, this is where a lot of activities have taken place at the Death Race.

Corn Fed Spartans - An obstacle racing team that started in the Midwest as primarily a Spartan Race focused team and became one of the larger obstacle racing teams.

DNF - an expression often used in a variety of racing communities to denote a race that was not finished, for whatever reason, you "DNF'd" or otherwise you "Did Not Finish"

Death Race - An ultra endurance event held originally in the Green Mountains of Pittsfield, Vermont. What started as a part of an ultra marathon under the Peak Races banner back in 2005 evolved into the tip of the spear event for what is the now global, Spartan Race, which was first started by Joe De Sena and Andy Weinberg.

Hercules Hoist - The Hercules Hoist is an obstacle with a rope attached to a large weight or stone that is fed through a pulley 20 to 30-feet above the ground. The participant must hoist the weight to the top of the pulley system and slowly lower it back to the ground without dropping it.

Original General Store - This is one of the best and is kind of the only store in Pittsfield, VT. It's a place where Death Racers meet, greet, and eat. Many memories are made in this store, before and after this one of a kind event.

Riverside Farm - This is where Joe De Sena's event venue exists, it's located on a beautiful piece of land next to a river and backs up to a mountain with dozens of trails to explore. Many operations for Spartan and Death Race began and operated out of here.

Shrek's Cabin - Located at the top of Joe's Mountain, this is a cabin that over the years has been transformed by Death Racers, during the race, or in training when people have stayed with Joe to better prepare themselves for the event. Many hands have gone into building this iconic Death Race cabin that often serves as a checkpoint during the event.

SISU - is a Finnish concept described as stoic determination, tenacity of purpose, grit, bravery, resilience, and hardiness and is held by Finns themselves to express their national character. It is generally considered not to have a literal equivalent in English.

Spartan Race - Spartan Race is a series of obstacle races of varying distance and difficulty ranging from 3 miles to marathon distances. The series includes the Spartan Sprint, the Spartan Super, the Spartan Beast, and the Spartan Ultra.

Spartan Endurance - the branch of Spartan Race that I developed during my time as a Spartan employee. Spartan Endurance consists of non-distance based team and individual events that include the Hurricane Heat, the HH12HR (a 12-Hour Hurricane Heat), and the Agoge.

Team SISU - an endurance community and team that started in California that has grown across the United States but still has it's team base primarily located out of California and the Western states.

The Suck - Unofficial slang term used by the Marine Corps. Defines any situation in and around a war time conflict where conditions are undesirable. Also known as "The Shit." We faced manufactured undesirable conditions in an effort to better ourselves and see what we could endure, to see what we were made of.

White Barn - The White Barn is located on Riverside Farm and is often used as a checkpoint location for the Death Race, it's also used as a cabin for wedding events hosted at Riverside Farm.

WHAT AM I UP TO TODAY?

It should go without saying, but my story isn't the only *Legend of the Death Race*. I continue to share the legends of other Death Racers on the Legend of the Death Race podcast and you can subscribe on most streaming platforms. Check it out at www.legendofthedeathrace.com. I hope you'll tune in weekly to hear more legends!

Currently, I am happily living in Seattle, WA and enjoying all the natural beauty this city and state has to offer. Most of my weekends are spent running up and down the various mountains throughout the great state of Washington, rain or shine!

Exploring volcanoes, mountains, and various peaks has become my true passion, and I have the Death Race to thank for introducing me to that lifestyle.

I am also working on my next book, still in the early stages, which involves a plethora of conversations with endurance athletes and a lot of research into what motivates humans to test themselves in such grueling activities.

If you would like to keep up with my current adventures and for information on my next book, you can find me at www.ThatEnduranceGuy.com. I'm also on Instagram as @ThatEnduranceGuy. I share information on those domains about all the races, adventures, and gear that I encounter or create.

What about Race Director Life?

I'm still directing races, currently I am working on the SISU 24 Ultra PNW which is a 24-Hour Choose Your Own Adventure running event, where racers camp out, and run as many of the 5-6 trails we mark as they choose to complete. Each trail offers some sort of bonus objective, from tying knots and memorizing poems, to answering a trivia question or returning an egg uncracked. It's a fun adventure that gives people the opportunity to see how far they can push themselves. With the Choose Your Own Adventure format, it's entirely in the racers hands where they go and what they see.

In addition to the SISU 24 Ultra PNW which I create in collaboration with SISU Endurance, I am working on some of my own race projects that are in the developmental phase. If you want to know more about what races I create, visit www.ThatEnduranceGuy.com to join my mailing list and you'll be the first to know!

I hope to meet you at an event soon!

Cheers,

Tony Matesi

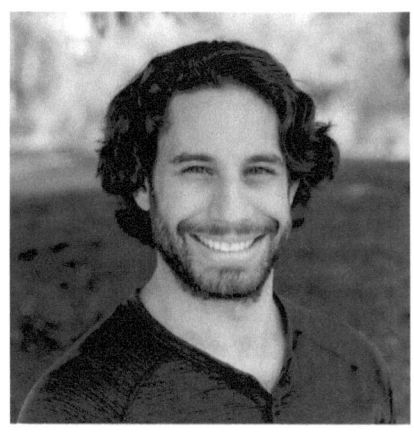

About the Author

Tony Matesi began his entrepreneurial career at the age of eight, copying and selling CDs and PlayStation games on the school bus. Since then, his passion for innovation has led to a unique career as an endurance athlete, sportswriter, and digital marketing professional.

From developing a cheerleading clothing line to building an international endurance event, Tony has always had a knack for finding niches and elevating them with his creativity.

As a lifelong athlete, Tony prioritizes health and wellbeing above all else and created the blog "The Legend of the Death Race" as a resource for Obstacle Race Training. Tony constantly seeks the next challenge and has competed at elite levels in Tae Kwon Do; gymnastics; competitive cheerleading; obstacle, endurance, and adventure racing; ultramarathons; and spent ten years on stage performing as a lead ballet dancer in the Chicago Festival Ballet rendition of the Nutcracker. He has competed in three Spartan Death Races, placed 3rd at the San Diego Alpha Warrior, made it to the City Finals on American Ninja Warrior, created a Death Race training program, helped open the gym REACH Fieldhouse in Chicago, launched Spartan Endurance Internationally and brought the ultramarathon event SISU 24 Ultra to the Pacific Northwest.

He has dedicated his life to helping others and has been a life coach for peers, consultant to global businesses, and used his athletic expertise to help motivate others to achieve their dreams.

Even though this is Tony's first published book, it is not his first published work. As the former Editor in Chief of **SPARTAN Magazine**, Tony's work has been shared and printed in various publications in the world of obstacle and adventure racing.

He continues to update the Legend of the Death Race blog with new podcasts each week that share the "legends" of other Death Racers weekly. You can find out more at www.legendofthedeathrace.com.

Tony continues to blog about his latest adventures in mountaineering, ultrarunning, and all other things endurance on www.ThatEnduranceGuy.com.

Thanks for reading!

If you enjoyed this book, please consider leaving an honest review on your favorite platform.

www.ingramcontent.com/pod-product-compliance
Lightning Source LLC
Chambersburg PA
CBHW031059080526
44587CB00011B/749